A Final Examination

The Doctor Looks Back

Scott –
enjoyed the music
at Williams – hope to
see you again, hopefully
under similar !

Robert M. Taylor MD

ISBN-13: 9781492278085
ISBN-10: 1492278084

TABLE OF CONTENTS

FOREWORD

It was early summer 2012 and Cindy and I were traveling in Scotland for the wedding of a godchild and had the opportunity to make an impromptu sweep about the coast of the old sod, traveling as we enjoy doing with a wandering vagabond style, let whatever will happen next happen. We had done a similar trip 25 years earlier heading directly and deeply into the fabled Western Highlands, savoring the awesome Isles of Mull and Skye, unforgettably so but necessarily leaving the east of Scotland undiscovered as if expendable, which on our current journey we were finding not at all to be the case, enrapt in the architectural treasures of Dundee, the grand history and decorum of St. Andrews, even industrial Aberdeen unveiling wonders. Scotland's own trove of the medieval, castles and king's trappings, substantially consolidated in the Northeast.

At any rate it was on such a non-itineraried Sunday afternoon that we impulsively took a turn off the high coastal highway of the far Northeast from which the lofty views of the tumultuous North Sea lack nothing, a signpost indicating a 1 kilometer descent into what was likely to be a quaint fishing village which promised a brief and perhaps interesting diversion. Never be afraid to peel another layer of the onion. We did indeed find such at the water's edge, a coarse craggy shore with a mere couple of rows of ageless stone cottages mostly in attachment with each other. Not a soul in sight, the windows shuttered, curtains drawn. Silence prevailed other than the bluster of the wind rolling in which substantially opaqued the weak sunlight bravely attempting to penetrate. We were drawn closer to the water's edge by another even more primitive weather worn structure with a dilapidated dock protruding a matter of feet into the angry sea. The tiny irregular windows were all either sealed with centuries of layered grime or off-kiltered but firmly hammered boards. On closer inspection we were excited to find on the upper outer corner of the landside exterior a bronze plaque -deeply tarnished, wind and wet damaged, installed at the roofline which was barely at eye level in the ancient way.

We were able to make out something about the British Historical Commission blah blah and with a light rub with the sweatshirt sleeve uncovered the inscription, "On the day, August 23, 1908, on this site (still rubbing), absolutely nothing happened." In retrospect I am quite certain behind each of those curtained village windows lurked a very entertained Scotsperson having a hearty if introverted Sunday afternoon guffaw.

This story, admittedly extraneous but still fun to tell does, however, segue into the question of why in the dead of winter, now 2013, it began to nag at me that I needed to compose a memoir.

My name is Robert Michael Taylor, always has been, Robert because Thomas had been ruled out as bad luck after the tragic motor vehicle death of an unrelated Thomas Taylor, two weeks before my birth September 30, 1947 in Elyria, Ohio; my father Alexander Taylor was in search of an "American sounding name". Despite the fact that he was derived from a long line of Alexander Taylors, all beholden for survival to the coal mines of Dundee, now long since closed down; he apparently had experienced since his own arrival on this shore at the age of three a Scottish sounding appellation to be somewhat burdensome.

Around here, the burg of Pittsfield, Berkshire County, Massachusetts which has now been home to my wife and me for a quad of decades, I am also known as Dr. Taylor. Or variously " the doctor", "doc", "Dr.Bob", "Dr.T", and other such including probably a more derogatory under the breath or behind the back designation at times perhaps by a disgruntled patient unappreciative of my assessment or recommendations. They do say "don't shoot the messenger."

At any rate I have been doing my work for a long time. I am a family doctor. I have been doing it long enough that now nary a day passes without the question arising as to when am I not going to be doing it. I do not know the answer to that question. But I do know that when I think on the matter or have the same chat with my also venerating colleagues, that I, alone in solitude or we in community know that when we cease our professional efforts we are not going to be replaced.

That is an issue over which I have considerable remorse. I am of the opinion that when our ship sails into the sunset, taking the practice of family medicine with it, our way of life, our culture, and our social identity will be the lesser for it. I believe that what takes place between a doctor and a patient can strike a level of significance that rises into the sacred sphere. I do expend energy grieving the imminent demise of my profession (Say it ain't so, Joe), but actually not nearly as much as it might induce in that I have chosen to put such energy into coming to understand why I carry that feeling so powerfully, i.e. what is it that is being lost. Did something of value happen here? Something worthy of a plaque. Or not.

A long way of saying that it has occurred that taking a look back at my own trials and travails might be a good thing to do, perhaps just for my own purposes, perhaps also some thoughts and memories that my dearest family might consider adding with pride and some curiosity to the family record. Give it a place on the shelf. Sort of kind of like that. I mean why in the hell did the Neanderthals go to all that trouble to paint those awesome artistic renderings of their own lives on those cave walls. I am told that those caves had no electrical outlets even to plug their word processors into, never mind the absence of an espresso maker at hand.

So I digress. Yes I digress. But I am not in a hurry. I am at an age where I don't do much fast and soon I will in fact have more time on my hands than I have had for half a century. And likewise eventually a major chill. So no need to rush. Why not make a few notes.

Perhaps not without coincidence as I wrote these few paragraphs, from my second floor study room, which looks down on our Wendell Avenue roadway, a UPS truck just pulled up allowing its driver to extract from his vehicle a cardboard shell presumably containing an electric Yamaha P-155 piano and dutifully place it on our over-sized porch which stands directly beneath where I am sitting, writing and look-ing out. Sort of fun to sit and reflect while watching someone else working. It occurs. I once read that Hemingway only wrote in the standing position. But if he really drank as much as history reports, could he really stand that well for so long? But again I digress.

A warning and a promise to the reader. If you do not appreciate or cannot deal with this vernacular approach to the printed page, Stop Here. I subscribe to the Mark Twain school of thought on that - "Why use a 25 cent word when a nickel word will do just as well." I am also way too old to take a course in writing or any other new pursuit really. Do rest assured on the other hand that whatever is reported herein falls under the trusty umbrella of the truth, naturally a relative phenomenon in and of itself. Fear not, friends, family, patients (it occurs to me as I write that, how inter-changeable those three domains have been in my life), fear not in that I really have very few axes to grind. They have been ground.

Addendum: If you want the real truth inside the truth, you will have to read the poems. They are the vessel which holds that which was otherwise too difficult or painful to express.

1

A CALLING

LET'S START WITH a library scene.

    Libraries have always been special places for me. The quietude of the library suits me though the value of amplified noise has not escaped me altogether either. My predilection for libraries I believe has more to do with being surrounded by banks of books. My early childhood was not without its stresses, I'll get to that, but I do remember getting a warm and fuzzy feeling entering the children's division of the Elyria Public Library, say 1953, with a kindergartner's eyes, being taken by the massive number of books and even more so by the little oak boxes of numbered file cards which I learned could speed your access to the right book for you at the time. Hats off I thought to Mr. Dewey and the entire decimal construct both of which appealed in concert to my already developing sense of order that the whole of life could be reduced to the right letters and the right numbers, but they did have to be the right ones, and in the right order.

    The room seemed cavernous to me though probably was no bigger than our current living room. Definitely miniscule in comparison to the University of Michigan Graduate Library with its volumes measured in tons and megabytes. An awesome library twelve floors into the sky and open 24 hours, my kind of library. We will get to that.

Parenthetically if someone would be so kind as to Facebook me a recommendation on how to write a memoir without the incessant use of "I," "in hindsight,' "upon reflection," and "as I recall," etc. I would be greatly in your debt.

The library in question at the moment, however, was located in Pittsfield, Massachusetts, on the second floor of St. Luke's Hospital, rather buried in an obscure corner alcove that had probably been little used for an eon or two, also fairly diminutive like the children's reading room but definitely less utilized. The hospital itself was heavily embossed with yellowing prints of the Virgin Mary and the Holy Family with statuettes of Jesus on the Cross arrayed on most available horizontal surfaces, plenty of possible shrine sites in case a sudden need for a diffuse community prayer broke out. Virginity otherwise was not enjoying a major run in the said environs in the early 1970's. I do remember watching the Watergate congressional trials while I was there, Sam Ervin making John Dean's hairline recede even faster and all. We did get rid of Nixon shortly thereafter so someone must have been going to church. The library was more of a heavily set thick oak motif of tables and chairs and a lot of Home Depot type slatted painted blue steel shelves (foreshadowing the imminently arriving Home Depot).

We have jumped to the summer of 1972.

I am doing a medical rotation at Berkshire Medical Center, the St. Luke's Hospital being one of two sites along with the erstwhile Pittsfield General Hospital, the two recently merged. It worked out as Berkshire Health Systems now has about 40 subsidiaries and care facilities in about as many states as Thomas Jefferson purchased calling it all Louisiana. It was not an exhausting rotation by the standards of the time. Making rounds in the morning, some time writing charts (we were still in the hay day of carefree rainforest decimation), a not hurried free luncheon in a small cafeteria packed with starchy white uniforms of every description, a welcome to St. Luke's workup of a scheduled admission or two, (the idea of scheduling a medical admission is now totally quaint), allowing a reasonably paced individual to luxuriate in the library until what I learned they called in New England "quittin' time." Old St. Luke's was a great place to develop an appreciation for several generations of Italian immigrants without which a serious consideration of ever practicing medicine here would be misguided.

On one such day sitting at one of the four library tables claiming most of this library's square footage, probably keeping my head aloft with a precisely strutted forearm (we did have muchos night call at that time and were in a continuous state of sleep deprivation), I happened to spot a few feet away a moderately thick but ancient well-worn book with a royal blue oilcloth cover and a finger nail polish insignia of title and Dewey enumeration. The re-covering had to have been the work of an enthusiastic and probably damnation fearing volunteer matron of the church, maybe even a nun, on the endangered species list at the time. The Table of Contents interested me as apparently this volume was the autobiography of a country physician who much earlier in the century had gone into medical practice in a small town in northern Vermont and stayed the course of fifty years on his job. This amazed me. Each of the many chapters was dedicated basically to some spectrum of pathologies.

This random picking up of a dusty volume (I recall that the insert withdrawal registration page had been vacant) occurred at a time when our country was in the demoralizing, paralyzing morass of the wickedness of our Viet Nam dalliance which ended up with 58,195 of the names of my generation carved into The Wall in Washington. Those were the ones who came from the wrong side of the tracks, or who drew too low of an LBJ draft number, or who were unprotected by a medical school student deferment. Few in my generation had gotten past the fear of a general disintegration of our society into a state of chaos to worry about getting any kind of a work situation in what we called the straight world (now has a different meaning) or anywhere close to the Establishment. I was also typical of the period in time in that I had a stated desire to practice my trade somewhere where people really needed me, where I could make a proverbial difference, amusing to me now as I would soon learn that such a noble effort could be acted upon truly anywhere and at any time of one's choosing. Nevertheless, fate had played a hand. This crusty old treatise of medical recollections from the other half of the century, probably written by some retiring but never to retire wizened Yankee doctor dressed in a seriously worn if not tattered woolen suit having a difficult time with seeing the cataract refracted light at the end of the tunnel with nostalgia and discomfort, looking for a way to say adios amigos, had worked as a potion on this emotionally vulnerable, morally confused, not yet committed, (but should have been committed somewhere) fledgling hippie doctor in cowboy boots.

I was hooked.

2

CHILDHOOD AKA BASIC TRAINING I AM BORN.

WHETHER I SHALL turn out to be the hero of my own life, or whether that station will be held by anybody else, these pages must show.

(I long ago concluded upon reading any number of memoirs, that if one is going to plagiarize, one should do so flagrantly and with verve.)

My sense is that given the goal of these writings is to dig down into a life given over to medicine that the years of growing up can be given a quick gloss. That was, however, also my presumption upon embarking on four decades prior some weekly counseling/therapy sessions that would rapidly metastasize into a steady date for several years. It came more naturally to Sherlock Holmes that one must return to the scene of the crime.

To begin my life with the beginning of my life, I record that I was born on September 30, 1947, reportedly a beautiful autumnal equinox of a day, by my own calculation an exact 280 days (the human gestation), after the preceding celebratory welcoming of the New Year in that fully stoked era of post-war baby booming. This in contradistinction to the September 23, 1981 birth of my fourth daughter Emily Catherine on what I can more personally verify as a consummately beautifully foliaged autumn day here in the Berkshire Mountains, in fact the same interval of 280 days since the preceding celebration of the eve of Christmas. All occurring under the watchful gaze of the same unmoving Star of David. Amazing the coincidences in nature.

The next three years is a definite blank.

When I took my leave of those premises another fourteen years later with my accumulated possessions - assorted jeans, shirts, a toothbrush, and a short stack of Beatle albums - in the trunk of the family's Chevrolet Belair, chauffeured by my father, much more anxious than I to get off to Ann Arbor in pursuit of higher education. The first in our line to have that opportunity. I also took with me what I perceived to be fairly happy memories of a fairly happy childhood, in a fairly happy town in the northernmost of a fairly happy state, situated a mere toss from the gently rolling waters of Lake Erie. Unfortunately those waters had shifted in chromaticity during my growing up years from a vibrant aqua blue to a sordid murky rustiness (Benjamin Moore might say Fecal Brown) which metaphorically echoed the flagging of the American dream as it stretched its Superman Cape from VE Day and VJ Day across the domain of Ozzie and Harriet to the opening acts of our foray into the rice paddies of Viet Nam and our inevitable loss of innocence, also echoing my own.

What can I say about my childhood?

I liked baseball a lot. Still do. My first professional ballgame was attended at age seven at Cleveland's own Municipal Stadium, now returned to the earth, but then cavernously able to accommodate 75,000 with an expanse of green that massaged the imagination of fans young and old. The status of our busload sentenced us to outer upper deck left field which on that day conveyed the benefit of watching the visiting Boston Red Sox leftfielder, Ted Williams patrol the territory for 18 innings. This was still the era of doubleheaders - miraculously equaling only about five quick no screwing around hours - or about the amount of time reserved for beer commercials in a televised contemporary American League nine inning game . What I do remember but have never seen since is the resplendent epitome of the same Mr. Williams' body unraveling like a corkscrew in an explosion of fused strength and grace as he took a swing aimed for the right field fence. Herodotus indeed.

I remember having in my pocket an actual George Washington dollar bill which was enough to make the purchase of right there in the concrete aisle three hot dogs and two pops (in New England, sodas.) I also remember seeing with my own eyes Vic Wertz who in 1954 hit the ball that Willie Mays caught, Bobby Avila who in 1954 hit .341 to lead the American League, Larry Doby in centerfield, the first African American to play in the American League, whose fleetness of foot in center and power at the plate enthralled the young eye much more than his skin tone, power hitting catcher Jim Hegan, whose failure to appear for the second game, replaced by Hal Narragon, disappointed. It was explained to me that catching at this level was so arduous that two games in one day was too much. Not in the old days I thought and if I made it to the majors as a catcher I would most assuredly catch both games. My kind of a job really. Though my true passion had already become shortstop in the center of everything happening and also if gifted with good enough of a glove one's agent could make a better case for a lesser hitting performance which was in fact consistent with my own skill set at the plate, though I could lay down a bunt with precision. I do not remember who won the game that day other than one very happy little boy from Elyria and about 74,999 other Little Leaguers and their dads.

I also remember back on the Little League bus being positively stimulated by the height of the municipal architecture of downtown Cleveland, (That's the Terminal Tower!!) and also finding the collected aromaticity of the fumes of many buses not unpleasant, the fragrance which I would later learn to be the remains of diesel fuel combusted. The love of all things urban has nevertheless never left me.

My home life must need be addressed but as much later investigation would repeatedly demonstrate what I do not remember has always overshadowed what I do remember and I was more not there than there. My father was substantially absent from the domicile more literally, committed to his professional endeavors for very long hours, what he would refer to in his retirement years as "his career" grinding out a living for the five of us (I have an older and a younger sister), trying to perfect the Moen single valve faucet. He spent those years saving every possible farthing of his proceeds as exampled by many generations of his Scottish forbearers, for eventually educating his progeny or whatever rainy day or old age might require, a mindset of prudence that growing of age through the American Great Depression had greatly fostered. This was in considerable opposition to the more luxurious streets that I assume his parents dreamed of when they packed a steamer trunk and sailed to these shores, my father en tow in 1924.

My father carried within him a forest fire fueled by a large reserve of ambition, anger, resentment, determination, jealousy, shame. Scarlet O'Hara on steroids. He had been immigrant depression poor and wanted better but never really found a way to leave the humilities of the past behind in that his feelings for his native family and culture also included a profound depth of love and respect for all that precluded such a transition. Thus a man capable of intense feelings, sentiment, and love came to be largely sacrificed upon an altar of internal conflagration. Not without considerable collateral damage. He was to find great soul soothing and the necessary dose of forgiveness in the faithful practice of a medium right version of fundamental Christianity which kindly reinforced his own needs to feel holy. In any case my father's personality qualities made his very early and very late work hours, i.e. his absence, not a hindrance to the maintenance of a reasonably stable domestic tranquility in our household.

My mother's presence was more invisible similar to the demeanor which also served her children seeking safety near the fires of my father's intensity. She was my mother. Marie. Same name as my third daughter Marie Susan and her daughter Rose Marie, (nine months of age at this writing). She and my father were lifetime lovers being early childhood neighbors in Amherst, Ohio, both family's residing on the same lane in modest rented houses, drafty and creaky I am sure, built to be within walking distance of the nearby sandstone quarries especially convenient for the times when there was work. In those backyards they both learned a love of gardening, the nobility of earthy root vegetables, which was both joy and necessity during those years for survival. Anorexia nervosa had not yet been culturally popularized. Hunger had. My mother's was a household of three in that she had no siblings, and often two as her childhood was punctuated in capitals by the bitter reality of my grandfather's alcoholism which created a bloodbath of a childhood for my mother and necessitating many long term stays with her father's extended Roman Catholic family of siblings "down home" near the Chesapeake Bay.

Frannie, Michael (my middle name, patron saint of Protectors), Theresa, Mary, Margaret, Katie, and William. No kidding. My mom's mother (Catherine) had not yet become Grannie B., patron saint of my family, and she had no siblings of her own. Her older brother had died from tetanus as she was growing to adulthood at the century's turn "down on the farm," the only child of a Cork, Ireland, mother and her German husband (known in Amherst as "the Kraut") in a state of desertion from the Kaiser's army and seeking a safer landing zone a more comfortable distance from the German magistrates, this in an era of very short trials. I have often and long been deeply thankful for the Kraut's slice of the Germanic being added to my otherwise bivalency of Scotch and Irish, imbued as it was with an affective fieriness a little hot to handle. None of the three DNA ethnic cords stood in the way of agility with numbers.

My grandfather's alcoholism was the prevailing wind of my mother's entire life endowing her with an inability to ever dream of asking for much never mind what she deserved. I will never forget the tears on her face during a conversation years later at a time when she was suffering with some depression of her own as she confessed that she would have wanted to go to college too. Probably at the time not even a consideration as she went into the factory directly after Amherst High School to manufacture parts for fighter planes for the war effort. She read fiction incessantly for the whole of life, mostly alternative reality type of writings - family dramas, romance, travel. I never saw her indulge in any form of alcohol until she much later would occasionally take a sip of perhaps a teaspoon of some very sweet sherry to be polite on a holiday, a culinary choice which probably would have served her only son as a wiser alternative to his own choices in that area.

Suffice it to summarize that my mother was a wonderful if oppressed woman, intellectually gifted if oppressed, and full of love and pride despite the same oppression for each of her three children. I will be forever in her debt for the steady and continuous blanket of support upon which my childhood was acted out. Regardless of the lofty height at which my father would set the bar, my mother was always able to counterbalance with comforting arms communicating that I was pretty okay as I was. I recall one dark rainy day in late October returning home from my elementary school with a report card in my slicker laden with a B, my first of the same, in fear of losing my status of paternal immunity and my life in general being over and my mother holding me and telling me it was okay as I cried buckets and that maybe that it would be a great time to get working on my Zorro costume for Halloween which we then went to her sewing machine and skipped supper in order to finish.

Key to the psychoanalytic dynamic which all of the above implies it must be included that I grew up also within walking or two-wheel bike distance of all four of my grandparents and both of those homes were at least equal to my own in terms of formative effects. From about age five, I was free to roam. My own recollections of 147 Fairlawn Avenue and 336 Harvard Avenue on which my father made mortgage payments is more of a vague sense of not really ever being fully present, an ethereal void, as opposed to the warm feeling of generosity and comfort at home with both Grandma and Grandpa Taylor and Grandma and Grandpa Bradley wherein I was treated like royalty, fully tutored on the ways of the old country and the old days, taught a salivating taste for the ethnic dishes (my eye still goes to fish and chips on any menu), allowed to offer my own theories and responded to in kind with their accumulated wisdoms. They were all much younger at the time than I am now but I owe to them my relative sanity, whatever aspects of my personality are tolerable, and my deep appreciation of the value in life of being able to both laugh and cry, sometimes simultaneously. They read to me, taught me the Bible, threw the ball to me, cheered for me, picked me up and dropped me off, in every possible way. I owe them everything. They especially taught me that whatever deficits I might have to cope with at home from the parenting of my parents it must not be too bad as they both came from these four and somehow all had managed and survived.

Thank you Grandma Kate for the uncountable number of plates of Scottish pancakes, the great joy in my life which Fish and Chips have brought to me, the wonderful story of your first date with my grandfather Chay when you had Fish and Chips from a paper cone strolling the main street in Cowdenbeath village in 1918 and then my grandfather farted "just like a Taylor" and that it was oh so okay to fall in love in life and occasionally also to fart.

Thank you Charlie for being my inspiration, my role model, my North Star for what it means to be a man, that great strength can be clothed in great humility, that in the love of a woman lies the ultimate meaning in life, and that believing in God transcends all else. Thank you for encouraging me as a boy to one day "hang up my shingle" which from this vantage I realize was enough to make all of the finger bleeding sacrifices you made for your family across your own hard years somehow worthwhile.

Thank you Grannie B. For being such a force for the value of awesomeness in the world, the absolute epitome of grace under pressure, for letting me park on your lawn, for making me know that you wouldn't even be angry if I parked the Chevy on your porch perched on the swinging bench, for making me bologna sandwiches at five in the morning to take caddying, and I am definitely glad that you didn't die after I yanked your long hair after you yanked my long hair - hey what's this- and we both laughed so hard and couldn't stop that I was certain one of us was going to have a stroke and I wasn't sure which.

And you need to know that when I raced over to your house when you called me to come quickly at 11:30 on that Saturday night and my parents were out and I rushed in breathlessly and saw you sitting alone at the end of the couch under the soft golden incandescence of a single bulb looking like a fallen angel, making the room all quiet and transfigured and you told me that grandpa had died downtown of a heart attack after a meeting and I held your hand and comforted you with the pained silence of loss on your face with the tears of having loved a good man for a lifetime welled in your eyes was the moment that I knew that in my lifetime I could really help people in a special way which I had never before dreamed of and that that was the moment when I decided to be a doctor.

And thank you Grandpa B, John, I loved it when your friends called you Jack. Thank you for never missing my games. It took my daughter Amy to have a baby boy, Cullen Alexander, a generation later to begin to understand the adoration that I always saw in your eyes when you looked at me. Thanks for the dollar you gave me for playing the piano at the birthday party, it bought a whole pile of baseball cards. And for the Timex watch on my birthday and the electric football game on Christmas. And the socks on my sister's birthday. Thank you for implanting in my soul an insurrectable knowledge that no transgression cannot be undone by an honest forgiveness and commitment to change, that it is both noble to forgive yourself and to be generous in the forgiveness of others. That we all live under the grace granted by a higher power.

I have never offered a treatment to a patient, roused during the night to go to a bedside, offered precisely the right word to set in motion a state of healing, placed my hand on a patient to share and alleviate some manner of suffering when you were not breathing and present in my mind, my heart, and my soul.

To all of these people I say thank you.

And I also had a friend. At grade level 3 in Miss Eggert's classroom Bruce and I met, and soon took a mutual oath of blood brotherhood to share the whole of life's promised discoveries. In the early years this included passages like our first phone call with a girl, our first dances, our first dates, personal research on the facts of life, many more ballgames, first sleeping on the beach, our first can of beer. The Beatles concert at Municipal Stadium was epochal. My first bar mitzvah, his very own, my first visit to a temple and an evening of a proud Jewish family's idea of gala, very new to me but an immersion into the world of the Judaic which I have never ceased to find kindred. We lived an inseparable childhood and I also found a portion of my needed refuge in his household where there was a parental void, both Barbara and Marvin putting in extraordinary business hours in pursuit of the coinage necessary to gala at times, pretty much leaving the joint to Bruce and I to kick back. I remember from that abode being impressed that the black and white television was somehow embedded in the wall, there was a chess board in the living room with quartz players situated on a marble table which never left their appointed squares, and Bruce's personal shower door was embossed with a pulchritudinous silhouette that made bathing seem a less mundane waste of time.

We were soul mates, saw the world the same way, shared the same slightly macabre sense of humor, both were bloodhounds for hypocrisy and bullshit in general. Holden Caulfield as Siamese multidenominational twins. We helped each other find ways to navigate the straits of what the world would inevitably require from each of us. We would ultimately attend in tandem the University of Michigan Medical School, both emigrate now with our brides to New England for further training, both found what would become large medical group practices here in Pittsfield in our respective specialties. Bruce and Reba and Cindy and I have now been neighbors for close to thirty years living in classic New England gentry homes which in both of our childhoods would only have been mansions to dream upon. There is now one house sitting between us which I can only hope discourages any amateur psychologists from suggesting an excessive interdependency.

Our lives have been largely lived in parallel as we have each been busy ministering to the townfolk and raising four children each, all eight of our progeny knowing, however, that they had backup parents at hand. Given the primacy of our long and enduring marriages, it was otherwise to each other that we have always turned in times of most desperate loss. Having Bruce to hold me in his arms the day Amy's friend and soul mate Sylvie was killed by a drunk driver as I tried to hold my children in my own weakened arms can never be repaid. In June of 2012 it was my own honor to officiate at the wedding of Bruce's oldest daughter and Peace Corps veteran, human being extraordinaire Meghan and her New Zealand husband Paul, neither of whom were interested in a rabbi or a priest. Another first for us. It is good in life for someone to have your back.

How any of this played into an entering into the medical profession remains problematic. I do remember in kindergarten when instructed to draw a picture of me when I'm grownup I crayoned a desk and a stick figure, hopefully with a kindly face, and labeled it Doctor Taylor. I had learned letters and words a couple of years earlier trying to figure out the comics.

I also remember occasional home visits from Dr. Robinson to assess we three kids and pronounce which it was we had - the measles, the mumps, or the chicken pox. I think I wondered why I didn't know anyone else who had the first name doctor. I remember the same Dr. Robinson doing a pretty brief physical and filling out a form pronouncing me fit for being an undergraduate student at the University of Michigan about a decade later. He was a man of few words but did seem kind and reassuring. I remember being proud that he was the President of the local Medical Society though in hindsight I am certain that was a position won by default. I imagine when I indicated to him an interest in medical school that he thought to himself a "good luck with that buddy, you don't know what you're getting yourself into."

More unfortunately I also remember having a succession of "wheezing attacks" that tended to last the whole of the nocturnal hours for the two weeks our family spent for vacations at East Harbor State Park, sleeping in the cool dank of a rapidly aging fungal-ridden canvas tent which for comfort was pitched on a scattered fifty cent bale of hay purchased en route for the purpose. In subsequent years I came to realize that as a child I was a fairly serious asthmatic that any number of those nights could have been fatal events and what were my parents thinking. The ultimate solution was for me to wheeze and sleep in the car which was a welcome improvement. Was the fiscal sensibility of these camping vacations, the fun and frolic on the Lake Erie beach, really a reasonable parental choice? Could my executive father not afford or envision a motel type of vacation? Go figure. It did constitute good early training for the enduring of interminable nights.

I do remember some vacations visiting my mother's Irish side of the family on the Chesapeake shore with all those Irish eyes smiling, delicious Down Yankee accents, colorful songs and laughters in the air, the waft of a local lager or two, hearts bursting with family affection. I remember how much my usually more stern father clearly loved these people and happily joined in the fracas. Not to detract at all from the Tiffin Sunday afternoons spent hearthside with the Taylors with the curious aroma of the pipe pervading, 40 winks for all before it was time for tea and the re-heating of the Sunday dinner remains along with opening of canned corned beef and some canned fruit and vegetables put aside in the larder from the largess of the remote summer toiled over garden by the blessing of the Lord. These were truly strong, deep, thoughtful, loving, reserved, hardworking, remarkable first generations folks. But even at the age of seven the afternoon's requisition of four words per person spread out over seven hours seemed a bit austere.

I remember more cogently sitting in the corner barber shop with several buddies and Dan Nixon the barber, also our go-to source on sex education, after school one day about grade 7 when a dapper gentlemen with an exceptionally white shirt entered, sat in the chair, got trimmed by Dan, throughout the clipper and scissoring service immediately drifting into and remaining in a deep sleep, then rising, saying a quick thanks, and leaving as if fully recharged. I asked Dan who was that and he responded, oh, that was Dr. Shork, a name of consequence to me as both revered and legendary in our community as the first and for many years the only practitioner of the art of obstetrics in my hometown, and provider of such services times three to my own mother including on September 30, 1947. I remember being captivated by wondering how could a grown adult possibly be that bone tired, that in need of a nap, for what cause would any adult so willingly accept a life spent in the throes of what appeared to me to be such a rapturous state of fatigue. There was a touch of glory and fulfillment in his countenance of expressionless self-knowledge I remember fully, knowing then and there that that state of consciousness was something that I wanted for myself, with a passion. I did not know at the time that life would fulfill that desire so imminently nor so completely.

Piano Lessons

"Yes is the answer,
and you know that for sure."

Mind Games
John Lennon

"There are two things Impossible to get in the Vatican.
Honesty and a good cup of coffee."

Pope John Paul I

September 1953.
I am six years old.
I am a first grade student at Garford School,
where I arrive daily at 8:25a.m. for the first bell
with two Lincoln pennies
submerged in my dungaree pockets
for milk packed in a yellow carton dropped mysteriously
from a blue a vending machine
a long two hours later.

On Saturdays with equal punctuality at nine a.m.
I ascend the dusty staircase of Day's Hardware
wearing out of respect
the same scuffed Buster Brown school shoes
to an unknown cavernous forest of unnumbered rooms,
my own destination populated by an ancient upright,
an oak bench which parallels the horizontal

of my polo shirted abdomen,
a straightbacked chair and its occupant,
known to me as Mrs. Bemis,
whose frail and pale dermis
is amply immersed in cotton and tweed,
a woman who touches me with her cold, spiny fingers
only to mold my own tiny fingers over the worn ivory keys
with kindness and patience,
a weekly ritual carried out in return for one U.S. dollar from my parents,
transporting me from Every Good Boy Does Fine
over the ramparts to Swan on the Lake
crescendoing past Ten little Indians
and on to the Marine's Hymn
with which a year later I am able to elicit
a smiling approval from the usually stern Mrs. Schoolcraft
in the Garford auditorium.
I remember from all of this that middle C occupies
a special locus on the written music sheet midway between the upper and lower clefs
pierced by a short horizontal axis all of its own
and likewise is the centerpiece of the keyboard
unique unto itself.
It seemed a safe harbor to me,
at least one unit of centrality
which might remain a coefficient of constancy
for the storms and machinations which were to come.

Thelonius Monk was born on October 10, 1917,
to a family immersed in the dusty hopelessness of poverty
in a rural North Carolina village known as Rocky Mountain.

His mother was taken aback when she overheard her shy and awkward six year old
rhapsodizing melodiously on an out of tune country church piano;
the family determined to migrate to the Big Apple
where the child remained self-taught,

performed professionally at age twelve at Harlem rent parties
and proceeded to codify the harmonics which came to be known as bebop,
with his left hand cruising from stride, through bebop,
and into the Land of Modem Jazz like Marco Polo
with rocking and lurching rhythms of his own design
as he created his own musical universe,
cadences dropping through unseen holes like Alice in Wonderland.
The world of piano was annointed with a new before and after.

I was next to sit on a bench in front of the 88 keys two decades later,
childhood blurred by like a single random wave broken upon the shore,
my new instrument a traveled Lenox Village Kluet upright
rolled down church hill on casters,
bestowed by the angel who had come to live at my side
who thought I might like to play.
I was a husband now, and a father, and a doctor as well
unfazed by whatever clouds which mightwant to gather.
My responsibilities seemed manageable.
Middle C had remained in its same spot.
I played daily
extrapolating from that center note
a succession of immediate possibilites up and down,
very interesting - it was really all just math.
Lessons seemed like a good idea,
the standard approach really,
despite my generally orthodoxed compulsion
to insist on wheels only of my own making
at pain of death;
at that age I was my own reference.
The lessons ceased rather abruptly shortly thereafter
as Michael's hand,
which I had previously admired
managing the lower span of the keyboard
with great facility

rested greedily upon my inner thigh
as my own hands were anxiously searching for correct notes,
the startling revulsion of that grip aborting my attempt at trust,
seeming to confirm my addiction to the exclusivity of my own paths.
Fortunately some years thereafter the fear
of a repeated concertina of sexual panic
was bypassed by the need for incipient pianist Elizabeth
to have her interest sweetened by a parental co-sufferer.

Harriet, erstwhile concert pianist in her far gone youth,
was to be an experience to cherish.
Safely distanced need by her advanced chronology and patience of manner,
the withered waterfall photo taped on the wall at the grand piano's flank
said simply "Things Take Time."
This proved correct as she guided me through scales and some Schubert and Haydn,
confirming for always my love of this process.
Sadly that partnership came to a shortlived conclusion,
as her many decades nurtured thirst for dry vermouth,
a predilection which my teacher and I did not altogether not share in common
reaped its toll on her aging liver,
and she became my patient until a much too soon demise was reckoned,
her kindness to me exchanged for
my kindness to her,
in a field of endeavor much more natural to me, doctoring.
I remember her fondly
and her orphaned music library
has since been subject to my protectorship.

Jason Moran was born in Houston, Texas, on January 21, 1975.
He began piano lessons at age six but is said to have longed to quit
until being exposed to the recordings of Thelonius Monk.
The rest was to be an irreversible lasered trajectory
to the outer limits of his craft,
still only now a just beginning journey;

in the darkened sanctuary of the Village Vanguard
I first experienced his genius as he was only barely out of childhood,
attacking and enveloping the Steinway with warp speed tenacity,
a mellow sonority, an unleashed explosion of virtuosity,
seemingly received from out of the Other but followed by
the humble referential explanation as some work
that he was exploring with His Teacher.
Oh My.
His teacher.
That would be the Buddha? Ludwig Beethoven? Amadeus? Bach?
The prodigy explained
that all music was simply derived
from the work of those gone before
with some simple additions and refinements.
Thus the Pantheon.
The Duke.
Art Tatum.
Fats Waller.
Count Basie.
Bud Powell.
Horace Silver.
McCoy Tyner.
Herbie Hancock.
Chick Corea.
Keith Jarrett,
possibly the single most significant pianist of the jazz years.
Dr. Billy Taylor.
Kenny Barron.
Marcus Roberts.
George Shearing.
Errol Gamer.
Madam Marion McPartland, elegant and wonderful.
Mulgrew Miller.
Eric Reed.
Junior Mance.

Brad Mehldau.
Kenny Burrell.
Professor Oscar Peterson, genius of the romantic.
Ahmad Jamal.
Cecil Taylor.
George Cable.
Hilton R uiz, Nuyorican mystic, left hand from heaven.
Renee Rosnes.
Eliane Elias.
Bill Evans,
who believed he lacked talent and "had a confidence problem,"
but proceeded to re-define the chord voicings of modern jazz,
the consummate master of nuance.
Harold Mabern,
at 70 too busy being a student to consider himself a teacher,
who believes that if you are worried about making mistakes
rather taking challenges
you might as well just sit down.
Sitting down being a strategy
which I have never been inclined to embrace.
Oh there have been passing moments,
growing up being life's constant temptation.
I have borne witness to every manner of abuse, violations, desertions;
heart-searing losses,
untimely deaths,
agonizing physical pain,
impoverishments of spirit,
the despair of depression,
tragic injustices,
evil assassinations,
senseless rejections.
Perhaps my most difficult lesson
has been that treachery in the long run
is most likely to appear out of the hazy mist
from the most unlikely and unexpected of purveyors;

beware the wolf in sheep's clothing,
the wise man bearing gifts,
the snake oil sales man,
the silver tongued con artist;
and that to find truth,
the ultimate reality is that the ugliness
which must be the first to be stared down and consumed
is most likely to emanate from one's own heart
There are no saints.
There are no sinners.
What does exist in this human journey
is an infinite complexity of choices
from which each of us must
finally mold our ultimate fate
just as the pianist sitting before the constellation of keys
in the silent moment of prelude before playing
faces an array of choice that is unwritten, undetermined.
From these masters I have learned this greater reality.
That there exists for us mere mortals an untapped wealth
of luxurious insight and awakening;
that the spectrum of our lives can be decorated
with glorious beauties and perfections,
of limitless possibilities for good.

It is midnight in the darkness of Birdland.
This stage is sacred space, an altar,
previously trod by the greats,
Miles, Parker, Coltrane, Getz;
Bill Charlap is seated before his nine foot Boesendorf,
the instrument intertwined as if in love with its perfect mate,
its perfect partner, attended to by its own maestro,
a grand duet.
An acre of piano.
A piano Field of Dreams.
The song is a ballad, an aged composition from the Bird,

which the players proceed to climb aboard like pilots on a fighter jet,
to ignite fires, to strangle, to extort,
to cajole, to weep over, to prostate and pray over,
to worship, and to plead with,
for what seems an inexhaustible duration
gradually easing toward the making of peace,
a slow triumphant head bowed march to the sea,
slowly embracing the concept of resolution,
accepting that a final note must become inevitable,
and then caressing that final holy tone.
Prince Charming kissing the pure lips of a sleeping, fallen angel.
I am in awe,
in the prolonged moments of silence of collectively held respiration,

before the applause erupts,
I am a fortunate wayfaring spectator,
a student at the foot of the master,
recipient of secret knowlege,
my first ever awareness
that with all of our carnal limits,
there is such an entity,
that there will always be hope for,
that there will always be the possibility,
of a perfect ending.

"Anything, everything for der Kinder."
Bubbie Yarmosky

3

HIGHER EDUCATION

DEFINITELY AT TIMES, we were a little high, but relapsing into lifting Dickensian phraseology, "It was the best of times and the worst of times."

On the last weekend in August 1965, at which time my entire wardrobe and the bulk or my earthly possessions could be easily accommodated by a graduation present suitcase, my father and I took the drive down the Ohio Turnpike, took a turn North on U.S. 23 and an hour later were driving down Washtenaw Avenue and onto the University of Michigan campus. The only other items I remember taking with me were a semester of college credits from high school and my Beatle records which I still have but don't travel with as religiously. I had never been in Ann Arbor or that many places at all for that matter. My destination was Room 401 Allen-Rumsey Hall, soon to be renamed 401 Ballyard, a dorm room assigned to me by some University housing officer whose job in the current must be greatly simplified with the advent of modern computer technology.

This landing was of far greater gravitas for my father than myself in that this was a dream fulfillment for him having carved out a successful professional life on the wings of a high school education and mountains of hard work in order to one day be dropping his only son off at college. I would be the beneficiary of the advantages not on the table for himself at the same age.

Myself, I had no idea what I was getting into. Just that this was next in line for what one does in life, following a logical sequence begun by my parents handing me over to Miss Short at Garford School for kindergarten. My guidance counselor had felt this to be an appropriate academic environment for me. I do remember being awed by the idea of separate buildings the size of my old high school reserved for each discipline, being able to root for the Wolverines as if they were my team just as the Pioneers of Elyria High School had been my team. I liked the idea that I could come and go entirely as I saw fit even though my coming of age years had never lacked freedom.

At any rate after stashing my suitcase in the dorm my father took me to lunch upon the completion of which I excused myself to empty the contents of my stomach in the closest men's room. Unless there was something wrong with the tuna fish, the butterflies must have been less ready for my emancipation than I was cognitively aware of. My father took back to the highway about twenty minutes later. It don't remember the parting being sentimental in any manner though the recollection of the first drop-off at college of my four daughters years later comes back to me with vivid, agonizing existential clarity. That sense of your chance of doing everything you can for your child being over coming down like a sledgehammer with brute force, magnified by the deepest love for this child, the high water mark of your life's efforts. Ouch. Grotesque in its finality.

I don't remember my father expressing any of that; neither do I remember asking him to hang for a while. All I remember was that after I puked I felt fine.

It was moot a couple of days later when after standing in block long lines to enroll in classes, a task also likely greatly simplified since then by modern data management, it was back to the classroom, to study very similar subjects to my high school curriculum, just geared up a little, taught by teachers using much loftier vocabulary and significantly more animated gesticulation, and swimming in a deep end of high school valedictorians.

Back in the dorm it did not take long for the sobering fact to sink in that I was one sliced onion in a stew of pre-med student minions, for the largest part prepped, groomed, and bar mitzvah in various well to do Detroit suburbs, places unknown to me, sabers drawn for doing battle for coveted medical school admission. In my naiveté this was a new reality to me. Ironic to me fifty years later how difficult recruitment of young doctors hopefully wanting my job seems to be. At any rate the pressure seemed to abate considerably a month or so later when the scores of the first organic chemistry departmentals had been posted and half of the pre-med students promptly became pre-dental students.

For the next three years I took what I had to of hard sciences required for medical school but my main interest was in another area. I took every course I could in psychology, hammering away at a fundamental question which to this day I continue to struggle with - is the human brain an artist or a computer, is thought an electronic construct or ethereal maze, is human memory, personality, consciousness a system of neurochemical equations or the spiritual made manifest?

I remember being held over after class one afternoon by a particular psychology professor whose ideas were brilliantly inspiring, wanting to inquire about my plans after undergraduate studies. When I replied that I was headed to medical school, she offered an "Oh, what a waste!" which I knew was meant to be a compliment. My game plan set out in kindergarten was cast in stone, of course. I really had no idea what an academic career would look like but I still wonder at times if I had shown an interest that day in her invitation to come and talk about graduate psychology studies, perhaps sometime in my life I may have come across an idea or a treatment that would have made a difference in the world in a more general way than my many decades of the trench warfare one at a time ministering to the wounded. I do think that eventually I would have come up with one good original idea. On balance, the far greater truth has been that at that time I had actually not even begun to grasp either the soul level price that medicine would exact from me as a human being or the complexities of the intellectual and spiritual dilemmas to be analyzed and fought over. Even more fair to say that I had no basis on which to anticipate the magnitude of the gratification that would come to me from those efforts unwinding the mysteries and miseries of my kind, one never ending fascination. It has never been boring.

Two other factors from my undergraduate experience should be mentioned. The first is that while I was busy getting educated, Lyndon Baines Johnson was succeeding magnificently in converting a small was into The War, burying our national conscience and freedom loving identity in the rice paddies of Viet Nam, a debacle which would shape the ethos of my generation and still plays out to this day in the character of our national life. It is impossible to separate out from anyone in my generation the impact of that long, bloody morass, an experience we would take with us eventually re-shaping the American Dream. Every tradition, every social moray, every social value and construct would be called into question and altered in lightning force fashion never before seen. Much was gained, and much was sacrificed. History will have to measure which wind prevailed. In the words of Dylan, The Times They Are A'changin. True enough.

The other tidal event is considerably more pleasant to recall and happy to report. Late in my sophomore year I had been chilling with an old friend one Friday night quietly in my apartment, somewhat drifted off into delta wave when my roommates returned from some revelry somewhere, accompanied by some new friends fortunately all young women. From this vantage it is difficult to recall the full complement, but I will never forget, not for a moment, not to the end my first look upon one particular angel. I can place where she stood chatting, basking in the amber light, fantastically being herself. She was cute, pretty, and beautiful rolled into one. I can remember her expression which exuded a calm self-knowing with a willing and amiable openness, right and what is next. Rather ravishing in all ways. She was seventeen years old.

She did not notice me. Otherwise when I called her two days later to ask her out on a date, she would not have thought I was my roommate. When I picked her up three days later she was able to dismiss the confusion and we headed out to the movies. By the time we returned to her home at the end of the evening and several hours later than her parents thought appropriate we had covered a rather wide spectrum of what issues we thought important in modern civilization - art, politics, history, philosophy, psychology, religion, etc. - and had come to the conclusion that wherever our journeys might take us that we wanted to leave, travel and arrive together has held for the ensuing forty-six years. The miracle of that evening, the blessing of finding Cindy at my side for always, being anointed with the promise of one true love has always stood above all else in my life as surpassing understanding. In the words of Robert Frost, "And that has made all the difference." I was made whole. Enumerable the times when it made all the difference indeed.

4

MEDICAL SCHOOL

Teach a Man to Fish

So it was with my innate Type A plus sense of hurried pacing that coupling some advanced credits from high school and one summer's studies allowing me to meet this standard pre-medical requirements, collect a major in psychology, be pronounced a Bachelor of the Arts after three years, aged 20, and get on with Plan A, the study of medicine, my quest. I was only technically a bachelor at that time. Cindy and I were fairly continuously at each other's side, including her sitting in at my preceding year's undergraduate classes. Her preference for the intellectual spell cast by my senior honors professors especially in comparison to her own freshman have-to's fused well with her intrinsic adherence to a doctrine of personal adventure and freedom but did delay a bit her own matriculation. She was then and is now a lifetime learner. And was in between. Curiosity incarnate. If you disavow boredom, choose a passionate craver of knowledge as your Coat from the Cold.

My acceptance of admission to the University of Michigan Medical School (the Leaders and Best rah rah rah) disentangled me from the need for a change in housing plans. We were committed to staying in Ann Arbor for at least four more years. My housing plan arrangements were already complex enough as the spider's web of social relationships, the loosely defined morays of the time, the way in which days and nights often blended, and the magnetic field that resonated between Cindy and I all contributed to a patchwork quilt type of domestic habits. It was due to and in the time of such circumstances that I remember nevertheless as if it was yesterday pulling up to the curb at the University Hospital Medical Center, chauffeured by a beautiful young guardian angel who seemed to grasp my dream more easily than I could myself, as I was disembarking from her seriously gentrified Ford Falcon, turning to me as I opened the car door, handing me the recently Eli Lilly gifted black leather satchel, and saying so lovingly, "Well, here's your bag."

Similar to March 5, 1978 when I came downstairs in the early morning into our Cliffwood St. kitchen, also Cindy's conception, at the time nine months post conception with our third daughter, her face brightly diaphoretic, vigorously stirring batter in a huge hand thrown mixing bowl which we still own; when I questioned the object of her efforts, simply responding with a quietly determined anticipation, "Birthday Cake."

Some of these things take time to appreciate.

We kissed.

And I passed through the hallowed threshold.

My best recollection of the early days of Medical School mirrored the transition to college in general in that it was clearly a deeper end of the swimming pool. The academic capabilities of my fellow students, the expertise and professional eminence of the faculty, the depth of the eternally honored traditions of the institution were also exciting and motivating.

I do not remember this time around any pervasive sense of competition in the air. The prevailing attitude was that none of us including the approximately two dozen women among the 200 (a breakthrough at that time though now a more appropriate 50/50 proposition) would be there if not deemed able and worthy. What you made of the opportunity became a matter of the dictates and efforts of each individual

.

Funny to think back now that in those cavernous rooms of interminable eight hour lectures for an unending two years I was sitting with two hundred doctors, a rather elite crop of sardine human tape recording robot brains. That would not now be my dream recreation. A few did freak at the intensity of the experience and disappeared discreetly without fanfare. The interpersonal competition may have been off the table but the size and ardor of the body of knowledge to undergo ingestion and digestion was not short of mammoth.

One experience I suspect all former medical students can retrace did occur in week one, i.e. entering an anatomy lab for the first time and beginning the process of dissecting a human body with scissors and scalpel, the assignment being over a semester to identify, isolate, and name in Latin every muscle, every artery, every vein, every nerve, every insertion, every lobe, every bone, every subdivision of every gland, the heart, the brain, the lungs and liver, and a few that you had not been previously made aware of. In my case the uterus and ovaries, of an erstwhile member of your own human race who had offered up their body for such instructional purposes. This lab was prowled by a team of anatomy graduate students who would descend like gestapo at the morgue tables to grill each of us in intimidating detail on the progress of our learning. At the time the anatomy lab at Michigan was in the "Medical Science One" building which derived from the pre-Great War era and had ancient brick walls, high arching fenestrated windows, and stone tablet tables arrayed across the expansive interior. One did get the vibration of participating in a secretive time honored ritualized rite of Galenesque passage.

This process the years would prove was totally mandatory in order to one day place hands competently on living patients and accurately understand the inside happenings, examine and diagnose with skill and knowledge. The corpses were tagged with their real names. I forget the surname of mine though I recall that it was a Jewish name. Her first name was Clara. I thank her in the stratospheres with deep appreciation and sincerity on my own behalf and that of the patients I have been allowed to serve.

Medical school is a good place to learn public speaking.

A basic mandated skill for every specialty, every ward, every grand round is the Case Presentation, a very systematically defined, ordered synopsis of any given patient providing in a specifically structured form all the salient facts of that patient's case at a given point in time. Failure to do this properly can put a student at risk for something between humiliation and legal public castration. It was such a presentation that I was fortunately assigned on a Friday early in my Freshman year, a case of throat cancer, to be presented on Grand Rounds on Monday, allowing me the weekend to prepare. After fastidiously composing my recitation on 3 by 5 file cards fully utilizing my earlier attained workings of the Dewey Decimal System I only requested of Cindy four or five hundred dry runs. A long weekend. She was unbelievably patient. Imagine my chagrin when I entered the lecture theater on Monday to find about 4300 white coated doctors with ENT faculty perched in a line on the front row like vultures on a telegraph wire. Dr. Walter Work, Professor Emeritus, Professor Substantus, 125 years old seated magisterially in the center of all like God the Father of the Ears, the Nose, and the Throat. Christ, he wrote the fucking book.

Imagine my chagrin further when after being called first and upon walking with the most confident appearing ambience I could concoct being with a finger wave summonsed to the feet of Dr. Work.

I knew I really had nothing to confess though I was more than willingly contrite as I leaned before him as he motioned for me to do. I will never forget the gravel in his voice as he whispered in my ear while stealthily picking the file cards from my sweating palm, "Son, I really believe that anyone with two degrees should be able to talk for a few minutes without notes." Fuck me.

Well, I rattled it off like a tape recorded announcement you can hear at any airport or grocery store, just like he knew I would. As I walked back to my seat in the medical student cheap seat area, he handed me my cards casually, knowing that they were of no further value, and winked.

I had been taught a valuable lesson about myself, and also about how there is a rather large number of ways that a doctor can learn to be a teacher to another human being. And that teaching is not a lot different than healing.

Well, there are a lot of stories I could recite about medical school but maybe that's another book.

My daughter Elizabeth, an aspiring writer, kept an aphorism Scotch taped for years next to her toothpaste - "Writing is like giving birth to a piano."

Maybe you should just take my word that I in fact did in fact graduate and we'll move forward.

I want to get on with writing about being a doctor.

Becoming one was fun, interesting, emotionally and physically exhausting, and required a level of intransigent dedication. This is as it should be. If a given student is not willing to forge that stream, the chances of being up to taking care of real people in the real world is nada. Medical school is shrouded in the delusional haze that if you can just get past it everything will become easier. My experience is that it proved to be mere novitiate foreplay that one can later look back at with whimsical nostalgia.

By far the most memorable event of my four years was the Spring break weekend of my freshman year when someone had made the arrangements for a church wedding with a couple of hundred guests, families and friends, some more well known to me than others. I showed up, got tuxed, played the role of the groom. My grandfather and some close friends recited scriptures and poems. Cindy was beautiful in homemade white silk gown and I have no recollection of anything other than just being totally in my head with love for her and it was only her presence that captured my consciousness. I wanted our love to be free and clear, total. I remember as we got into her father's Oldsmobile a giggling haggle of matrons probably well into their late thirties or forties handing to us a jewelry box over adorned with ribbons which we opened as we drove away. It contained a handful of shiny silver screws with an explicit note of directions. Lol. Actually the ladies' sentiment was not that inappropriate. Cindy was 19. I was 21. Seventeen years later I discovered that she was not perfect in all ways, but in the final analysis there are more important things in life than a person getting addicted to Thirty Something and then ER when the other person is trying to sleep.

On our anniversary days, now up to 44, we sometime reminisce about our brief but passionate honeymoon. We did not know until the evening of the wedding that some friends had sprung for a night for us in the honeymoon suite of a swank local Ann Arbor high-rise hotel. Though our student housing apartment with its shiny linoleum floors and glossy photos of each of the Beatles which came in the White Album taped between the boards and bricks of the bookshelves did not lack for romantic ambience. I forget where we got the bricks and boards but I guarantee we did not pay for them. The hotel was great though and we slept in until nine or so after which in that we had not packed for the night we re-donned our tuxedo and wedding dress, I think she wore the dress, and swung by my former apartment to grab my books, whereupon we headed to the library for seven or eight hours studying for midterms. Probably that was when she realized what a romantic she had married.

We were incredibly happy to be married. That is when my real life started. Back to the apartment, our only real piece of furniture was a gorgeous black leather lounge chair, genuinely tasteful, which somehow Cindy had eeked out of her wages working at the local American Automobile Association. Three dollars the hour? The chair was to serve over the next number of years as comfortable sitting for eons of hours of study canvassing the span of the medical curriculum and quite a few hours of unscheduled nappings. It eventually was retied and heavily worn to the carriage house and disappeared at the time of some cleaning out years later. I would give a lot to sit in it for just five minutes today.

For the record may history note that my main idea when I headed off to medical school was to become an obstetrician The process of conception, fetal development, the birth process, the whole thing in its entirety was as compelling to me as anything in the natural world. The study of the anatomy of that process, the embryology, the physiology, the cardiovascular dynamics and all were only an avenue to get closer to the magnificence of the birth process, the miraculous nature of which I saw as a potential conduit to knowing the divine.

I immediately headed off to the obstetrical unit when my freshman studies allowed for that leap into the clinical. I had a joyous experience at Wayne County General Hospital, half way between Detroit and Ann Arbor, delivering tons of babies and felt that my life would be an endless ladder of delivering baby after baby. This was followed by the matching gynecology clinic component which left me uninspired.

Please not the same thing all day. Then on to Pediatrics where not having really been around children since I had been one (though I sort of skipped that course anyway) I proceeded to fully fall in love with children. So I thought maybe a Pediatrician. Then on to adult medicine where I made the life altering discovery that adults were just partially grown up children.

So at that point I knew I needed to have the whole enchilada. Along came an Austrian immigrant physician to the Ann Arbor environs super- hyper specialization swim, Dr. Michael Papo, indomitable force to pronounce to the establishment the future of medicine to be the new epic invention of Family Practice. In my senior year I had the privilege of working eight weeks side by side with Dr. Papo's associate, a true country physician, Dr. James Botsford, who I found to be smart, in touch, generally cool, with the program and doing a lot of good. I was sold. At the end of the eight weeks I offered him a little thought for the day volume with the inscription, "Thank you Dr. Botsford; the others taught me how to be a doctor. You taught me why." He took from about his collar and placed round my neck a cowboy style string tie with a polished stone which had been given to him by one of his favorite patients. It still hangs in my closet and I reflect on my respect for and gratitude to Dr. Jim Botsford when I see it.

One last recollection from medical school days.

This takes place on a high level floor of the Mott Children's Hospital in Ann Arbor, state of the art mega institution for the care of children with the most serious of everything. It is about midnight. I am sitting at the bedside of a delightful little boy, Victor Mihalek, who if he is still about, I am certain can still capture a heart with a single smile. Victor had suffered a Drano accident which should never have happened and earlier that day had his esophagus reconstructed by Dr. Otto Gago, University Professor of Thoracic Surgery, from Argentina, himself an immigrant if not a refugee. Are not we all? Young, brilliant, dashing, swaggering but robustly humored, Dr. Otto Gago. The halls were darkened. Silence prevailed. Life and death wafted. I heard the clicking of his boots down the hallway before I saw him, entering Victor's room, placing his index finger on Victor's forehead, tucking a Teddy Bear under Victor's arm, nodding and walking away, hopefully to sleep. I thought to my own very tired self, that's the kind of doctor I want to be.

OBLIVION

Jackson Browne

I want to know what became of the changes
we waited for love to bring.

Were they only the fitful dreams
of some greater awakening?

August 1969

Mr. Yin, meet Mr. Yang.

The freshman medical student,
uncut hair and bellbottoms waving in synchrony,
strides into the open wound of a general medical ward,
12 West Medical, University Hospital,
the only necessary badge required for entrance
being an M1 nametag and a starched white lab coat,
which listed to his left with the weight
of the well-thumbed Washington Manual secured in his hip pocket,
a primitive external memory chip,
or perhaps a six-shooter to complement the cowboy boots,
scuffling across the glossily sanitized ancient linoleum.

His assignment would be a Mr. Charles Raines,
the task an H. and P., the beginning doctor's first.

"Hi, I'm Dr. Taylor."

"You can't be a doctor."

A Final Examination

"Too young?"

"No, too married.
You're married,
(glancing at the glittering gold ring
recently affixed to the doctor's left 4th finger),
and doctors shouldn't be married.
They should be like priests
and just be married
to their jobs."

The medical student
knowing from the moments before perusal
of this surly gentleman's medical chart
that the left upper lobe of this patient's lung
was encumbered by a fungating, fimbriated, tentacled mass
that amounted to a fatal sentence and imminently so,
intuitively understood that such a sentence
could make anyone skeptical
as to the motives of any potential caregiver,
and decided to let the marital advisability issue pass.

And thus they spoke.

At length.

Charlie,
with his deeply-lined pocked face of ebony etched with
a world of cold outdoor nights and hot in the sun afternoons,
both bathed in and soothed by the same Thunderbird pint bottle elixir

and with his steel wool beard and hair,
a random act of nature,
proceeded to paint a panoramic version of his life's story,
in a rural Southern rumble of ebonic adjectives and adverbs
that would make Faulkner blush honky.

What he remembered of a sharecropper baby's childhood,
his early in life hopping of his first freight train outta that town,
and then an endless series of freight trains,
his never-seenumagin' family,
his own marriage to the road in all of its promises and vagaries.

The telling was done with not an iota of loss or bitterness or misgiving
but with a resigned aura of tranquility;
he described in a poetry of his own making
deep-throated yassah drawl notwithstanding,
a vision of the earth as he had seen it-
awakening to the wetness of honey-fragranced morning dew,
the ecstasy of the wimmins,
working in the fields, and on the docks,
with every manner of pick and shovel,
and the romance of the open heavens passing by,
high above the midnight special.

His last words to me were:

"Doc, all I ever wanted was,
when it was all over,
to be able to say,

LIFE,

I hadda me summa that."

They hugged.

The truth was that for the doctor
the rightfulness of his recent marriage
which had only been a social sanctioning
of the bond which he and his lover had forged
in the instants of their meeting,
this marriage, this total eclipse of souls,
this rightfulness was perhaps the only issue of surety in his purview,
as twelve stories below on the streets of Ann Arbor,
a stew of protest boiled continuously,
tectonic countershock
to the military bloodbath the government of his homeland
was simultaneously wreaking
upon a starving strip of Asian soil
fiercely ready to defend itself
against the concept of being colonized by any white man,
a civilization hardened by centuries of battles,
determined to defend at any cost
its own identity.

We are and will be Viet Nam.

The utter nightmare of the grotesque inferno
had served to galvanize a generation,
an international army -
such that agreement on this single issue,

the evil of this war,
created a sense that all other differences could be relegated
to the primacy of that singular agreement,
that it was only one world,
and that it was shrinking fast,
and that we needed to get along.

I think of this now
as I stroll,
alone for the moment,
but marching on line with minions,
a coalition of the willing,
as the President would say,
beneath the sacred passage of saffron-draped Christo Gates,
a 23 mile sinusoid arpeggioed tunnel of color
anointing this Central Park
which somewhere in time had become my home.

Decorated today to celebrate all of the distance which we have come,
all that we ever were,
once upon a time,
and a proffered vision of what we could become.

7500 Gates,
monument to the eye of the artist,
a sweeping declaration as to the ultimate possibility
of man being just to man.

The thought comes to me as I immerse myself
in the surrealistic righteous glory of the moment
as the city which I love sighs a final prayer of acceptance
as to the treachery of 9/11,
and swims its way toward forgiveness,
that even in the greatest moments of evil in my own years,
as the blood flowed wantonly through the swamps and estuaries of Viet Nam,

the blood of innocent peasant farmers, women and children,
mixing and congealing with the spilled blood of my own generation,
my teammates, and friends, and classmates,
all of this blood mingling in a nightmare of carnage,
that God even then had a hand,
that the courage and fortitude of that beleaguered people
marked a watershed in human history,
akin to the Angel Gabriel appearing before Mary in Annunciation,
salvation is to come,
that among those humble people God had found a manger
for freedom again to be born into,
the corporate monster turned back,
the monster dragon of the empire pierced in its heart,
the deity of money chopped, its head cut off.

I know this now
as I know that I will not live to see it,
though my children shall,
yet oh what joy and beauty I have known and seen,

the Cliffs of Moor with sun setting in the West,
palatial vistas of the Eiger in the high noon sun,
the apices of great cathedrals and masterpieces of immortal artists,
the peaceful rise of the sun on deserted ocean beaches,
love made by the sizzling hearth of fireplace
warming us against the frosty middle of the night
full moon lighting New England fields of freshly fallen snows,
so much good work done,
so much love made,
so much learned,
perhaps the greatest of all
my wife, my love,
who, Charlie, you need to know,
was the One who believed in me
during the times when I was unable to believe in myself,

giving birth,
to my four daughters,
new hope brought to the world,
four more souls created to carry love into a tired world,

as I know that in my generation,
we did give birth to a new order,
that the largesse of the earth will be shared,
that the planet's glories will be for all to share,
Viet Nam to Manhattan,
Ecuador to Sierra Leone,
Panama to Sri Lanka,
Chile to Uzbekistan,
arm in arm together in each other's embrace,
one world.

Mahatma Ghandi.

"We have enough,
if we each just take what we need."

Just as today we make this march,
just as we flow through these Gates,
as one flowing mass of humanity,
freshly oxygenated heme through the heart of this city.

The Book of Genesis

"Then Jacob awoke from his sleep and said,
"How awesome is this place.
This is the house of God
and these are the Gates of Heaven." "

And yes each moment of insight
must be awakened from in order
to return to the ebb and flow.

As each symphony must reach its final climax,
every poem its final period,
every prayer its amen,
may the poet in me simply add,
that one definition of purgatory might be
to have left and not to have said good-by,
and though I feel well and feel ready for the long run,
the time is coming when I can say
that I did what I came here to do,
and that I did want to say to Mr. Charles Raines,
whatever distant corner of Oblivion you are hopping a freight train in,
that one day I will join you,
that my friend Romeo Rupinski who was a railroad engineer has promised me a ride,
and that the three of us will ride up front together,
that Romeo's lungs will be as good as new too,
that the whistle will be yours to pull until your heart is content,
and that we will be equal and together and hungry only for love,
but for the time being know that, Charlie,
life is life, yes indeed,
and I have hadda me summa that.

for my friend Joe,
who left without saying goodbye,
but whose heart still beats in mine.

5

House Officer

MEDICINE IS A profession which attracts the academic elite from our nation's second-ary schools (those with the thickest glasses, the most tragic haircuts, the least likely to get a date, etc.) into four years of pre-medical college curriculum (a Sahara Desert of organic chemistry washed down by physics, washed down by the phylogenetic dry gulch of biology), followed by four years of medical school, a fascinating fact infested swamp of teeth gnashing, nail biting, sleep deprived, migrainous sludge, following which you are fully equipped to do nothing whatsoever.

At that point your childhood friends are driving around in shiny new cars, pass-ing out their business cards, and setting tee times for Sunday morning at the country club. Not to mention the pre-med dropouts who flunked organic chemistry and went to dental school and now were driving BMW's. I had to bring that up again. Actually I have absolutely nothing but the greatest respect for the dental profession and give our family dentist the greatest credit for the fact that I have only one missing tooth at this point despite the perpetual chomping on Tootsie Rolls as my chewing apparatus was doing its own maturational dance eons hence. I'm certain the dentists have a more scientific term for that developmental process. As far as modern orthodontia is con-cerned one can only dream that our society had come as far in the manufacture of soft drinks that don't continue to pollute successive generations of our national dentition as the dentists have come in pasting glistening smiles across the faces of our progeny.

At any rate it was an orange Pinto which Cindy used to drop me off at the Berkshire Medical Center drop-off circle on July 1, 1972 to once again disappear through arched doors for some more hallowed halls learning. The Pinto was a gift from my father who I suspect knew that Cindy and I were on a fairly tight budget and that our 1964 Dodge whose odometer had quit long before in the 189,000 range was probably not going to get us safely to Massachusetts. Though it had done yeoman's duty. The Pinto had been outfitted with a carseat and also transported Amy, now eight months old, giving me two people in my life that I hated to leave even for a moment, let alone the unending overnights and weekends of call. The song Darling Be Home Soon wafted in the air. When I was accompanied by Cindy, now a woman, and her towhead cherub for hospital cafeteria meals, my heart pulsated with pride. The old New England town quickly and easily fell in love with my wife, Amy, and eventually her three sisters yet to be. I still have patients reminisce to me about "when your wife brought the baby to the office." My babies are now quite busy taking their own babies to the pediatrician, the dentist, the ballgame, the movies, gymnastics, hockey, etc.

This time the exact destination was a congress of medical wards, newborn nurseries, operating suites, emergency units, delivery rooms, and as often as possible the hospital library, never mind the occasional opportunity to snag some shuteye in the house officer sleeping quarters. The austerity of these accommodations was considerably buffered by the heavily hanging reality that myriads of our childhood friends still were shouldering their weapons in Viet Nam and were sleeping in rice paddies. Still, there were a fair number of doobies being rolled in both hemispheres.

This embarkation had been preceded a few short months before by what at Michigan at least was a traditional hoot and holler free beer family fest at Bimbo's, a venerable Ann Arbor institution premised on Dixieland banjoes and peanuts in the shell, where the shells get swept up every couple of weeks or when greater than knee deep. The faculty's methodology is to get the graduating senior class as soused as possible so that when the internship matchings to hospitals coast to coast get announced no one really cares. Anesthesiology was a strong suit in Ann Arbor. The occasion was similar to but different than The LBJ fishbowl draft number selection which was more like Madame Lefarge holding court aside the guillotine.

Cindy and I were more or less expecting to hear the name "Springfield Hospital" pronounced as opposed to the "Berkshire Medical Center" called out. "Where is that again?" but were not disappointed when we heard the word Massachusetts. A previous summer's barnstorm across the state had made us more than anxious to get our very own "Don't blame me; I'm from Massachusetts" bumper sticker. Our pre-childbirth scouting trip left us with a yearning to return here, for all of the colleges, for the fully died in the wool Democratic predominance, for the ubiquitous Boston dialect, the Freedom Trail historical largesse, and Cape Cod with its beaches and fried clam aroma stretching as far as the eyes could see. Cindy had been traveling casting a six months of pregnancy shadow, a great pride to both of us, a load less cumbersome for me.

A short story. We did have a moment of homesickness maybe two days into our sojourn when nothing we saw seemed any different than anywhere else and we were getting lost a lot. We decided to break for a sandwich at a ye olde pub type of place in Amherst, to pout a little when a jovial guy who introduced himself as Bob Gill joined us in our booth smacking a cold pitcher on the table and asking, "Hey kids, where ya from?" We explained. He listened. His prompt response was

"Ya know what I would specialize in if I was a doctor? Definitely. Definitely. The Rectum." We had met our first New England colorful character. When the pitcher had been drained and he had taken the temperature of our getting colder feet, he said softly and firmly, "Let me showya somethin."

We hopped aboard his traveling salesman block long Oldsmobile and he gave us the tour de force of central Massachusetts - the colleges, the prep schools, the estates, the lakes, the parks and back to the pub. He should have worked for the Chamber of Commerce. We were curious when we received via the U.S. mail in December to follow a manila envelope containing a single item; a pink flannel Christmas stocking embroidered "Baby's First Christmas." Signed Bob Gill. That's how we ended up in Massachusetts.

It was an idyllic June which we were able to spend between Graduation Day and the BMC drop-off. We had made arrangements to make to purchase of a bungalow on Housatonic St., Lenox, the price even at the time astonishingly in the range of a good used car. Reminds me of a time about twenty years later after

Cindy and I had dined at the Carlyle Room and been entertained by the legendary Bobby Short performing his cabaret show and I commented that it was a great show even if it cost a bit more than my first house, completely cracking up some East side gentleman of means standing next to us waiting for his cashmere coat. If he had seen the house, he would only need shrug, seems fairly reasonable. We arrived ready to hose it out, which it needed, to paint top to bottom, which it needed and to set up housekeeping. 64 Housatonic. Still has a heartwarming ring to it. Once we installed a potbellied stove, painted a mural on the wall, hung barn boards from an abandoned local railroad trestle, bought a ten buck paperhanger's table for banquets, and propped up the kitchen drain with a soup can and some duct tape, we proceeded to have a blast.

The transition from med student to house officer was remarkably similar to that from kindergarten to fist, eighth to freshman etc. Though to quote Eliot in ET, "Hey, this is reality, Greg." We were no longer working on laboratory specimens or practice dummies. The patients were now real live usually walking, usually talking human beings. The obvious goal was to discover the panorama of ways in which the previous Mount Everest climb of information accumulation could be applied in an effective manner to comfort the afflicted and afflict the comfortable. This was a transition that I reveled in.

I remember with some nostalgia and fulfillment the sense of having arrived at the correct destination, being certain that my goals and decisions had been the correct ones, and that the future held for me the promise of great satisfaction, the opportunity to meaningfully serve. Being referred to as "doctor" was no longer a linguistic contrivance dropping the "in training" but a reality that conveyed respect but also carried the responsibility to perform like a pro when called upon.

This sense of arrival was intertwined with an even greater degree of physical and mental grind, early out of bed, late to bed, calls up out of bed at ungodly hours, blood all over the place, excretions of every sort spraying and flaying all over the place, no need to draw a picture. It was the entire spectrum of human physiology gone amuck with disease, infection, rupturings, collapsings, overloadings, fracturings that was the appointed enemy. Quite a war. The private physicians whose patients the house officer cared for generally stepped back and let us do their work for them gladly. Plus there was a steady diet of formal lectures, conferences, readings, researchings, study to be concomitantly assimilated.

Cindy and I have now been listening to jazz for some four decades. We did have a second honeymoon after completing the freshman year, a brief if prophetic jaunt to New York City both of us drawn like a magnetic to the city where our karmas have never ceased star crossing. As recommended in the New York on Five Dollars a Day manual, we stayed in the upper upper West Side at the then Paris Hotel on upper upper West End Avenue which happened to be around the corner from The West End, a Columbia dive which at that time happened to have killer jazz nightly. Who knew. I love it when a plan comes together. Just so happened. We were just looking for a peaceful end to our evenings. What we found has lasted a lifetime. Last night by chance we ate some jambalaya and grooved on a virtuoso set at Smoke - piano, sax, drums, base (all it takes). Smoke, our Home away from home is around the corner, a stone's throw from the gone by Paris Hotel and The West End.

The more things change the more they stay the same.

It remains the case, however, that one builds an understanding and an appreciation of jazz as one might construct a brick wall, one brick at a time. When we stumbled upon the West End we heard two saxes, bass and drums, sans keyboard. Before that my knowledge of jazz was that I knew who Dave Brubeck was and an old college roommate from Long Island sort of worshiped him. After the West End we knew that jazz was its own universe and like the universe seemed to have infinite beginnings and endings. It was capable of re-defining infinity. Since then we have been experiencing jazz performances ceaselessly. One cannot say listening to or watching. It requires both and more. Experiencing in sensory fashion but also processing spiritually, using every level of your awareness. We have had the privilege of up close and personal with all of the great living jazz practitioners and have never seen two identical shows. In fact it would be hard to say we have seen two similar shows. Yet we have never seen a show that did not add to the foundation which would enhance and open the doors of enchantment offered by the next show. I have never felt that the full treatment can be duplicated at home with even the best recordings or for that matter in the perfect acoustics of a refined concert hall. Jazz at Lincoln Center has the Rose Concert Hall where millions of dollars were spent on ultimization of acoustic perfection. Give me

Dizzy's across the hall. Great jazz requires a room. As well as the dark, in the room as well as in yourself, as well as an inextinguishable ray of light with which to rekindle a ray of hope in the world.

A long way to say that becoming a doctor is like listening to jazz. One patient at a time you enter a room with a chart or a clipboard, a stethoscope over your shoulder, introduce yourself, ask questions, tap and press, think, feel, analyze and try to offer some understanding, some reassurance, some hope. And one room at a time you come to realize how infinite is the process and as you come to know less and less you become a better and better doctor.

Thus was advanced training.

Another memory from Housatonic St. It is something like one a.m. and we are sound asleep. If I am sleeping at home then I was likely awake in the hospital the night before. We have two babies of our own now, Amy and Elizabeth sleeping in their cribs. The phone rings, which requires a trip down the narrow staircase from our careful not to bang your head sleeping quarters. I am startled to alertness but shocked at the in a state of panic hyperventilating voice of an acquaintance from around the corner close to our same age: "Come quick, my wife is having a baby." It was obvious that he meant that second. I answered in rapid-fire that I did not do obstetrics but let me help him get an ambulance pronto, as in 911. I went back to bed and slept restlessly, a form of sleep that I would relive countless times in years to come, trying to find rest while pondering over the outcome of what had been recommended.

The following day I awoke with a sickened sensation and confronted an anger with myself that I carried heavily through the day and still can feel the ashes of. Why did I not just go? I love obstetrics! I am good at obstetrics! And I took an oath! A sacred oath. I felt a self-revulsion that I never wanted to feel again. Upon return from the hospital at the end of the day on the street I happened by the young man who had called in the wee hours. He was ecstatic, the proud father of a baby boy. He hugged me in gratitude, as I pledged in silence to next time deserve it.

I would soon learn that any mistake in the practice of medicine will always be shortly followed by an opportunity to try to do better.

It was a similar summer evening returning to our humble abode when Cindy mentioned to me rather casually as she was stirring a pot, "Oh, by the way, I bought a piano today." I am certain that my first question was for how much as I knew that our wall painting had left us with a single digit bank balance. "Forty dollars. I saw it on a file card at the Bookstore." Certainly seemed a bargain though I was still uncertain as to why we might want a piano. "Well you said you always regretted you quit piano lessons in third grade." How can you argue with logic with that? That night we rolled down the hill in Lenox an antique upright Kluett and found it a place in our living room. I have played almost every day since, we are talking more than forty years. For anyone accumulating a level of boredom with these writings, you could amuse yourself by keeping a tabulation on the number of ways in which loving impulses by the love of my life has changed things forever.

If you go diving for oysters, take along someone who knows what a pearl looks like.

Recollections of Housatonic St. would not be complete without the mention of Good Friend Coyote. Shortly after unpacking a circle of friends began to develop in our hood. Our best new friends were Janice and David, New York City drop-outs, who had tuned in and dropped out by opening a natural food store down the block. Friday nights became a regular outing night for this turned on network of friends to dance passionately in a circle to the rock/jazz/bluegrass/swing strains of Coyote. Tithe night was not complete until every one had taken a turn in the center of the circle. Some type of talk on the street system emerged - "Coyote's playin' tonight!!" and everyone would show up from out the hills. I will never forget the impromptu night of celebration at the roadhouse in Egremont the night Richard Nixon had proffered his resignation and waved goodbye, Coyote rocking out in a major way. It marked the end of an era. We were happy campers. It had been a time of great despair in the life of our society. All we had was the music but we used it to start again. Billy, Ricky, Dominick, Joseph, Pogo, Mark, I thank you on behalf of a Berkshire generation of young folks for being there when we really needed to have some fun. You were great.

I guess this is as good of time as any to return the same chair in the same St. Luke's library, once again sitting reading in the late afternoon, two years of medical training gone by. The volume Fifty Years a Country Doctor still shining lonesome blues from its shelf. I was slightly startled when Dr. Rubin entered, mostly because usually no one else at all ever wandered in. I was also a little startled by his directness when he half sat on the end on the library table and started with something like "I was wondering if you would like to join me in the practice of medicine." No sense spending a lot of time bull shitting around. I knew him very casually as I knew the entire roster of Pittsfield physicians. We agreed to meeting at his house that Saturday afternoon where Irv, Bob, Shirley and Cindy agreed to throw in their lots together. The rest is history and makes a good case for family being a matter of one's own choosing.

It is now time to be a real doctor.

DOCTORING

The beginning.
It is vaguely past midnight,
the quiet hours are upon us,
the tepidness of this summer Saturday night's revels
dissolving into a blanket of balmy quiet.
The squeaky gleam of the linoleum and the stainless steel decor
reset for another watch of readiness,
yesterday's misadventures, excesses, unexpectancies laid to rest
by this emergency room battle corps,
citizens by day,
a small city's answer to what might happen by the moon,
wordlessly communicating with grunts, sighs, sarcasms, exaggerations.

I am the captain of this ship -
though weeks before a green student and allowed to defer,
I am now the captain,
accepted as such by the members of this team, lifers in this town,
nurses, aides, orderlies with working class knowledge of life
not yet made room for in my child doctor's cranium
crowded with its lists, protocols, memorizations, graphics.

FIRE.

The tranquil winding down is shattered,
by the explosive racket of emergency,
adrenaline surges, the volume is cranked, and all hands are on deck
as Kevin and I leap through the ambulance doors screeching to the scene,
screaming sirened through the night to the conflagration,
clapboard dwelling belching smoke through its seams, out its doors and windows,
flames raging into the blackness of the night skies,

fire trucks strewn about, hoses lacing the lawns,
firefighters plying their trade with skilled deliberation,
sidewalks clustered with sleep shocked neighbors watching Hell.

There may be still a child on the second floor;
we vault the staircase into the mass of air thickened with swirling smoke
turn into the suspected sleeping place
blindly locate the child and find a pulse.

This I can do.

The blitz of breathing life into life commences
down the stairs, into the ambulance,
through the swinging open doors of the emergency suite, and into the night.
The patient is an innocent child
who hours before had pizza with her family,
watched a movie on TV with her brother and sister,
and before saying goodnight to her boyfriend on the phone,
had put on this Wendy nightgown and laid down on that bed,
and went to sleep and she deserves to live.

This was not to be.

For hours we compressed, injected, ventilated, bled, infused
in a sweaty tirade of refusal to allow, to allow her to pass,
to allow the reality that the cherry red coloration to her lips,
the dusky hope of whiteness in her skin
was merely the trademark signature of the carbon monoxide
suffocating her hemoglobin, stealing her life.
We stopped when we had nothing left to give.

I have often thought of that child.

Often on a summer night like that one
driving home in solitude from a bedside
enjoying the soothing chastity of the uncorrupted quietude
that abides when the living are taking their rest.
I wonder what life would have brought to her.
Children?
A loving husband?
Many Christmases and birthday candles and remembering anniversaries?

And I feel overwhelmingly fortunate about what life has brought to me.

The immense wealth of a passionate eternal love,
the glorious miracle journey of our four daughters,
and their own lovers, our sons;
the brilliant model of dedicated colleagues,
loyal and generous friendship,
so much of the earth exhibited so generously before our gaze,
so many gnawing truths revealed.

And the privilege of doctoring.

I remember that night and that girl, her life stolen,
and think how it was never going to be easy.

I could never have dreamed then
of the epic saga of human tribulation
that lay before me to put my hands to.

I would never have dreamed simply of the grueling expanse of the road.
The legions of the wounded, the ailing, the discomfited,
the self-absorbed, the self-abusive, the maligned,
the emotionally and physically violated.

The hours.
The many, many, hours.
The nauseated, the wretching, the hacking hoards;
the naive, the prevaricating, the loquacious spinners and sinners,
the talented naturals, the ingenious, the plodders, the malingering.

I would never have postulated the bizarre infinity of the narrations,
the stark factuality of the tales of this human family,
its grandness of fabulous masterings,
and equally legendary debaucheries.

I have been tole of mean street homicides,
maimed soldiers leaving parts behind,
sailors swash at sea,
parental and marital batterings,
infinite fidelity and rancorous infidelity,
addictions of mind, snortables,chuggables,
hatings and hurtings.

This required intense concentration,
carefully specific questions,
steady supportiveness.

And why do we do this.

Because no one of my patients
needs to be left to shoulder the load alone.

Because pain is among us, it is real,
and ongoing, and without limit
and deserves to be met
with the equal force of love and compassion.

Because I can.

Because even the greatest murky
desperate morass of hopelessness
can be confronted, can be engaged, understood, overcome,
when the hand of one human being,is taken ahold of by another
and led from the desert of isolation
to the open fields of rebirth, acceptance, peace.

Because miracles are miracles,
because miracles are for the asking,
and can be made the more plentiful
by opened eyes, an open heart.

Because it is for each of us to look into the eyes of the other,
and see the eyes of God,
and to join in the struggle,
wherever that struggle might lead.

It is late in the day now,
for that part of me
that wanted to answer that call,
that felt and answered that whisper of encouragement
in my soul to do so,
and perhaps now I have done most of what I can do,
came to do,
should have done,
but my heart takes a humble joy in reaching this point
more firmly convinced than ever
that there is grandeur in the fineness of the hand
that set me on the rightness of this journey,
knowing that when the end does come,
I will only feel loss over what could have been done,
not what I tried to do.

6

GET A LIFE

MY DECISION TO join Dr. Rubin was not greeted with universal applause. The training program which I had been in for two years was aimed at training internists though I had been modifying since medical school my own curriculum as precisely as possible to prepare for my own goal, family practice. As much emergency room, obstetrics, pediatrics as the program would allow. At that time there was considerable rivalry between the two disciplines. This hand to hand combat has disappeared over the ensuing decades as American medicine gradually evolved under enormous economic pressures and realities such that fewer and fewer wanted to do the work at all. The newer term primary care emerged and became the umbrella under which all first line of defense physicians tried to avoid the howlings of change. In the current time, you hardly hear the term internist very far off Park Avenue. And Family Practice, the shining star transitional object representing the modern evolution of the old time country doctor narrowly avoided crib death and is certainly having a stormy adolescence. At the moment it resembles a boxer bouncing off the ropes.

There are many reasons for this sequence of events. Most of them are economic.

One simple reality is that medical school costs a fortune. At the same time most medical students are paying for their own education and given the astronomic cost of undergraduate education, they and their parents have already achieved poverty. Thus the necessity of borrowing the tuition which costs a fortune, money made available by banks, government agencies, consortiums, etc. much like any drug dealer always glad to give a good client another fix. Thus upon graduation the doctor to be, generally a bright young person able to recognize bills coming due, is mandated to select a medical specialty that will likely pay lucratively. Favorites are plastic surgery, dermatology, ophthalmology, otorhinolaryngology, obthismonaonplatymegfailnitholgy, etc.

Another common ploy is to sort of screw the whole thing and work as a hospitalist or an emergency room physician (work a day, take a couple off) which avoids ever driving in a stake or planting a flag and rather fuses well with changes in work ethic and fading materialism which each generation takes its own vantage on.

Another factor in the equation is the infusion into the American medical legions what we refer to as the foreign medical graduate, who has been arriving on these shores in lofty numbers now for several generations. On an individual basis these people come here for the same reason anyone else comes here, for the same reason my grandfather came here. A better chance.

On a group level this phenomenon is a lot like the oil we take from the middle east, the art we steal from China, the sugar from Cuba which we consider to be our own - for a half century we have been and continue to allow third world countries to pay the ticket on the education of the medical professionals we need. Another subject.

The bottom line for primary care at this point in time is that most corners of primary care including the practice of family medicine are wilting on the vine. Doctors are very overworked, very underpaid (I don't try to make that case to schoolteachers, social workers, sanitation workers, people lacking green cards, the kid in the window at the Burger King or for the matter most of the human race other than liability lawyers and maxillofacial orthodontic surgeons.)

And I guess medical insurance company CEO's and Washington D.C. lobbyists. Not to bite the hand that feeds me.

The current era regardless of causation is characterized no one would argue by a downtrodden, often cynical, grumbling, whining gaggle of very exhausted docs who cannot help but question how did it come to this. Yes for society, but also for themselves. When they were young they were so bright and played so much by the rules and it all turned to such a mess. Pity. Welcome to the modern world is my take - who moved your cheese? Hello, you did. This is capitalism in action, this is democracy, this is a world with large numbers of people including some leaders who are more personally ambitious than overarchingly moral with limited resources to be distributed.

I once attended a Saturday New York Times public interview, an ongoing series for the Times.

On this occasion it was a pleasure to be in the same room with the operatic goddess Leontyne Price who openly told the remarkable story of her life. She reminisced upon her first arrival in New York City as a young student from the South, finding her room, meeting suave and sophisticated people, overwhelmed by the tall buildings, getting lost on the subway et al. In tearful frustration and homesick agony she called her mother from a payphone with her last dime. Her mother's response after listening patiently was a succinct, "Leontyne, get over yourself."

American medicine needs to get over itself.

To reiterate, I personally share in this sense of loss over the state of affairs we are immersed in.

I do fear for what is of lasting value to be lost in the rapidity of relentless change, somewhat of a regression to the mean, so manifest in every corner of our social milieu.

I also must say that I have never found the practice of medicine more fulfilling or more interesting. This does not surprise me as my life has been one of the counter-intuitive swim upstream but so be it.

This journey thus began with Irv suggesting, well why don't you come by about eight in the morning the day after the 4th. (That would be the fifth). Which I did. We then boarded his somewhat elongated gold Cadillac which could easily have accommodated another ten or twelve foreign medical graduates and we took off on a tour of the three local hospitals - St. Luke's, Pittsfield General, and Hillcrest Hospital. At each facility we would look in on half a dozen or so patients, each of whom Irv would greet with a smile returned affectionately, more often than not a hug. They could basically stay as long as they wanted which was probable good for everyone's economy. This would be followed by a short chat, scribbling a note on the chart (about six

words), and moving on, always ending at noon, time for lunch in the Hillcrest cafeteria. In the afternoons we would take turns seeing patients in the office, as our
quarters, the downstairs of an old house which his family occupied when he returned
a quarter century before to his native Pittsfield, cozy but not able to accommodate
both of us - 175 First St. This is a ritual which we proceeded to adhere to for several
years. We had a blast together, enjoying the personalities of our patients, discuss-
ing their medical details, talking some politics, being friends. This was very much a
father-son relationship for me and I still think on Irv often, in fact quote him in his
wisdom frequently and ask myself what would Irv do in a given situation.

We worked together for seven years. He passed away eight years later playing
a retirement round of golf in Florida with beloved grandson Robbie. I still visit his
wife Shirley hanging in at 95. If Irv in fact could see the hospital or the medical
office today, despite for his generation became amazingly adaptable and embracing of
change, he would be aghast. How could he not.

In a way I am glad that he did not live to see a medicine where you drop you
husband or wife off at the surgical center early in the morning to have some organ
removed and replaced and they tell you to keep the motor running, they will be back
shortly. Pretty soon you will definitely be able to lean out the window like at the
Dunkin Donuts and have your cataracts removed.

That was 175 First St. I still have patients remind me, "I've been your patient
since back on First St." with nostalgia of their own. We used to have a black and white
television in the waiting room and many were to locals who would wait for their consultation until a soap opera had finished. I remember one Sunday afternoon when Irv
and I, neither with billy goat genes crawled out on the roof to re-attach the angulated
antenna thinking that the sight must be curiously viewed by passersby as an interesting use of advanced medical training. Fortunately we did not end up in the bushes a
flight below or on the front page of the local paper, the Berkshire Eagle.

For whatever reasons - the amount of fun we were having, the pent up reser-
voir of medical needs accumulated by Dr. Rubin over 25 years of dedicated practice
needing tending to, the friendly smile and concerned welcoming to the office of the
delightful and gorgeous new receptionist (Cindy) - we were rapidly inundated with
patients. We usually finished the afternoon hours at about 6:30. Cindy and I had the

custom of a slice of lasagna or veal parm for $1.60 at a local spaghetti joint, The Rainbow, before home to relieve the babysitter. The patients loved it all, especially Cindy, only a little less so the doctors, and everybody loved The Rainbow. It was a grand time.

It only took a matter of months to realize that there was growth potential here and we began a recruitment process that has never ceased. The next year we interviewed a wiry young gentleman, New Jersey native, attended by his equally sincere and charming young wife, Suzanne. Suzanne was familiar with the nature of family practice as her father had practiced chiropractic out of her family home in Brooklyn as she grew to maturity. They both knew Ebbet's Field and the Polo Grounds and carried the worldly wisdom and sophistication of New Yalkers.

Suzanne came of age enrapt in the folk musical culture of Greenwich Village in the sixties and our conversation about greats songs, great lyrics, and great musicians has never waned. Sooner or later we are going play a song together. Gene was more oriented to the Mets, the Knicks, the Giants, though somehow he came to be afflicted with the same Red Sox and Patriots indoctrination which I have suffered with.

Gene and I rapidly found ourselves to be soul mates in the practice of medicine, fighting the good fight of making the world safe for family practice, the raising of a total of six brilliant daughters (count 'em), playing countless 18 hole rounds of golf in under three hours, and generally commiserating over every curveball and winning ticket life has had to throw at us. Brothers in Arms.

I would not have had the necessary persistence to doctor as long or as hard as I have without Eugene Heyman, M.D. at my side. When it was trench warfare he passed the ammunition. There is nothing we would not do for each other or each other's families. The days of arrival amongst of Ellie and Sara are held sacred in our heart - they are both out in the world now doing good work with tenacious commitment and belief in the ultimate goodness in mankind. Awesome children, the kind that you hand the world over to with confidence and delight.

The bitter reality of the dinosaur status of the work that Gene and I have done together, the image of a doctor to which we aspired and helped create has been a matter which we have processed jointly, arm in arm, heart to heart, supporting and encouraging each the other along the way.

Then along came Dr. Robert B. Lee very soon thereafter and we became RTHL, our custom at that time to just keep adding initials. Something like 35 years later his name remains at the same place on the list as he soldiers on. Bobby Lee as he tends to be known also has a roster of patients that date from his arrival, dedicated like crazy glue to the acceptance and trust they find in their physician. The key word here in this case is dry. Bob is a homozygous introvert. Some doctors wander onto the playing field of family practice because of outgoing, even jovial personalities, a natural ebullience.

In Bob's case my sense has always been because he does harbor a fascination with the machinations of the average Joe and his wife and children, as well as an appreciation of the rightness and dignity to be found in the common man. But don't expect to hear that from him. This is a guy who can finish work on Friday and reappear seamlessly at his desk Monday morning ready to work and respond to "How was your weekend?" with an almost under the breath, "Oh, it was good. I ran a marathon in London." And mean it. In fact that is a day's outing that he has indulged his 125 pound frame in very close to a sleek one hundred times. I'm not suppressing the exact number; it's just that he doesn't talk a lot. But that doesn't mean he doesn't have a quarter century of daily logs recording every run, the time, the ambient temperature, how many squirrels he saw etc. Still waters run deep.

Our group has the standard practice of periodic "business meetings" to hammer out policy, deal with political issues, manage personnel matters, talk money, etc. Currently this involves a consortium of eight partners All of whom know that the meeting is not over until I have pulled out the soapbox, pounded on the table, gesticulated in the air to the medical gods, quoted Winston Churchill, provided three historical metaphors, issued some thinly veiled threats, and run through at least a respectable gamut of profane vocabulary. I am not certain that these efforts are followed with a particularly sincere level of attention, i.e. as this is deservedly appreciated as who wants their rant quoted. On the other hand, an ole chestnut of an adage in our meetings has always been "When Bob Lee talks, everybody listens." His own batting average for finding the center of the nail being superb, he swings the bat only on select occasions.

And not long to follow, actually in tandem with Irv Rubin's retirement to the sunny skies of Florida, we were the beneficiaries of hitting the daily double. Out of the same training program in western New York Drs. Michael Murray and Jon Grenoble, bright eyed, dynamic, capable, wise beyond their years arrived in our welcome arms, welcome in that the growth of the practice remained unabated. The theory if we could just get one more doc we could keep up with things had given way to the reality that each new doctor had some type of parabolic effect creating a geometrically wider net.

In hindsight the arrival of Mike and Jon may have been the most singular event in the history of our group, giving us a core if I may say of five physicians with strong personalities, serious work ethic, a lot of charisma, able to develop on an individual level but also able to function with great group chemistry. Probably largely luck.

Michael Murray still can add, subtract, multiply, and divide faster and more accurately in his head and hit a golf ball with his trusty driver further into the sky than anyone I have ever met. Not always completely straight which compliments his interest in the biodynamics of the New England forest and also has promoted his being a doctor than playing on the PGA Tour. Interestingly he has a precocious daughter who sort of skipped elementary school and is at Tuft's Medical School at age twenty. His son Kevin also inherited his father's computational skills as well as his shoulders and I don't doubt will one day play tournament golf. And there is Randy, a Michael soulmate, signed on for the duration.

Jon Grenoble is what other doctors refer to respectfully as a doctor's doctor. As in what we all should aspire to be. Jon simple exudes competence in all spheres - an encyclopedia of medical facts on board, breathtaking facility at assimilating and integrating clinical information, innate sense of the vagaries of the human personality. The whole thing. Fortunately for Gene and I,

Jon also was blessed with professional managerial and business schools greatly relieving the two of us as we have approached our dotage with deftly assuming the day to day management of our practice.

Does Jon Grenoble have one enemy in the world? Not that I know of, frankly, other than perhaps himself. He sets the bar for excellence extremely high in every aspect of his life; I sometimes wonder whether inner peace and his kind of drive are mutually compatible. I am just glad that he sets more reasonable standards of performance for his associates like me. Regardless, I love him, as I do all of these guys, and would trust him with my life. He has two beautiful daughters of his own who both carry in every step the powerful deep and loving parenting given to them by Jon and his also brilliant wife Christine. Katie is now a graduate of the University of Vermont and bent on working on an international level to promote the wider dispersion of ethical and competent medical care, a grand design goal. A five minute conversation with her remarkable understated self would reveal that she means business. Sarah, younger sister, has different challenges being born with a corpus collosum defect impeding certain skills of cognition, but she also carries herself with Grenoble strength of character and continues to surpass expectations.

And there is Midge. Our first partner level female physician, and there are few like her. We have always set the goal of an ideal medical group being 50 % male/ female - this has been difficult in that while we have had a fair number of female doctors over the years, the exigencies of giving birth and raising children has tended to cause a preference for less than full-time workloads. I do not know the long term solution to that reality. I do know that it has been wonderful to have Midge in our practice to entrust with caring for my own four daughters over a span of many years, which she has done with comfort and caring, respect and discretion, a load off my mind. She's a great doctor.

Then of course the Kirbster, Dr. Craig Kirby, Desert Storm medical corps veteran which ironically provided uniquely appropriate training for our practice especially sharing a consultation room with yours truly for lo these many years. If Shakespeare was correct that brevity is the soul of wit then Craig's theory of practice has been if you say the say thing to a given patient fourteen times using different word selection each time maybe they will get it, an interesting thesis. Whether or not that is true I do know I would have gotten a lot more work done the last fifteen years if we had spent fewer hours trying to remember the lyrics of old rock and roll songs and sharing recipes together.

And there are many more.

The last few years, it has been a frequent occurrence for an aging World War Two veteran to confide a planned trip across the country somewhere to meet one last time with guys they were in the infantry with during the war, a half century before. A momentous journey but one which they seem to need to do before letting go.

I feel the same way toward all of my associates; we have been in a war together and have only survived by doing it together, protecting each other, supporting each other, sometimes taking a bullet for the other. These are great if unsung people. I hope that truth to emerge in the coming pages.

NEW YORK CITY

MARATHON

(1)

The Republicans are gone.
It is Friday early in the evening,
and they are off to the airports,
and they are gone.

This brings considerable relief,
the political equivalent of the street cleaners sweeping up in Spring.

The city can go back to being the city.

They have returned to their world of limp Wonder bread sandwiches,
      limp white organs between limp Wal-Mart sheets,
      de-sanitized lily white world of tea times and tee times,
      limp white excuses for their hatreds and jealousies.

And the wounds of terror,
which they came here to claim as justification,
for their violences, their armed devastations,
their bigoted massacres,
are now returned to us,
to our care and nurturance.

Color returns to the streets,
the tones of jazz pulsate once more,
conversation returns to its normal volumes,

animated opinions once again are voiced aloud;
we once again mingle and interweave
with acceptance and understanding
that the peace of the future
will be multi-colored, multi-languaged,
a tapestry of heritages.
We are the seed of that tapestry
as today we just begin again.

The towers will be re-elevated into the skies-
we will do this on our own time and in our own way-
and they will once again light the way to our city,
beacons of freedom, jubilant light.

(2)

"I can't wait to get back to New York City
where at least when I walk down the street,
no one ever hesitates to tell me exactly what they think of me."

Ani DiFranco

(3)

It is Monday mid-morning,
people are waiting,
on the 72nd St. train platform;
we are subterranean and en-route, awakening to the new week;

Her luminously orange dress is cut to reveal the entirety
of the lofty expanse of legs upon which she is constructed,
billboards,
giraffe legs elevated the more by spiked platforms,

facial features heavily painted for trade,
bushy headdress dyed, teased, blown to match the scanty garments;

and her counterpart stands dressed in the classic tarpaulon
of ancient achromatic Burkha;
femininity extinguished, no component parts revealed,

save for the darting out raccoon eyes and darkly pigmented sockets,
the cassock suggesting a robust if settled body form,
a life of silent intention, unspoken desires, untouched needs.

Polar disparities.

Yet they lean to each other,
approximate heads,
and converse in rapid-fire.

What information is so urgently conveyed?

Do they exchange recipes?
Personal opinions on pre-school curricula?
Who might be considered the best fifth grade teacher at the local elementary?
Neighborhood gossip?
Ideas on fashion trends??

Perhaps something about gender?
Perhaps the stereotyping, the marketing, the exploitation of women?
Something about the universality of male oppression, battering, sex slavery?
Oh, they have enough in common, things to talk about.

The C train rambles away into the darkness of its tunnel.
There are many more stops to be made,
passengers to be gathered,
synapses to be conjoined.

(4)

"I love, cherish, and respect women in my mind, in my heart, and in my soul.
This love of women is the soil in which my life is rooted.
It is the soil of our common life together.
My life grows out of this soil.
In any other soil, I would die."

Andrea Dworkin
June 28, 1975
Central Park, New York City

(5)

Winston Churchill

1900

"My opening lecture in New York
was under the auspices
of no less a personage than Mark Twain;
He was now very old and snow white,
and combined a noble air
with a most delightful style of conversation."

(6)

The marble bust of Ben,
in the full prescience of his maturity,
lips pursed with amazement, humor, a patient respect for our human condition,
my old friend, soul mate, mentor, cosmic support system,
stands but a few paces from the Temple of Dendur,
separated merely by heavy glass doors,
and perhaps an unseen grid of security wirings,

the lone remaining recorders of the nightly poker game of ideas,
which takes place,
after the guards in their institutional vestments have de-posted,
and scattered into the boroughs for the long and quiet solitude of the night.

What do they talk about,
these two, Ben and the pharaoh,
to carry them through the long celestial nocturnes in this hallowed hall?

How about them Sox?
Is the theater really dead?
Let's put on some Coltrane?
What's the closest place to get a decent bagel and a coffee this late at night?
Perhaps one of us should make a run to the French Roast.
How about we invite F. Scott Fitzgerald, Cole Porter, Eugene O'Neil, and Bill Faulkner
around on Friday night, crack a bottle of brandy and bang on the big questions?

(7)

We recline handsomely in our velvety box,
Cindy and I,
and Gilbert, the Music Man,
Janet and Albert, long traveled friends we,
happy enough in the moment.

The great walls of Carnegie echo with the holy utterances of musical deities.
Toscanini, Stern, Prokofiev, Caruso, Axe, Ozawa, Madame Leontyne,
have all in their turn suffused this temple
with what can be considered ultimate for those of our species
in our crying out for mercy from the gods.

Tonight, nearly four years into the new century,
we revel in the memory of a fabulous four musicians of our own generation.

Our temporal lobes retrieve the imprints of every incarnated gesture,
mouth with precision every stored lyric,
smile at every happy fragment of nostalgia drenching us.

These of course are not the Beatles.
Their names are Mark Benson, Gary Grimes, James Pou, and Greg George,
and they come from Akron, Ohio, and its environs,
and they have been doing this for 22 years.
Only James is able to play this gig without the benefit of a wig.

The creator of this magic carpet on which we fly, however,
the heart and soul of this explosion of creativity which still inhabits us,
the gentle artist of the soul,
who wrote all of these words of love for our own much pained generation
did live however for ten years of his life,
his final violently aborted ten years,
a ten minute stroll across the paths of the Park from this hall;
while he was at the Dakota
he was done with the gum chewing, and the witty sarcasms,
and the infuriated demands and protests for peace and justice;
he wanted only to live across from the Park,
to raise and be with his wife and child,
to feel love in his own life,
to be comfortable in his own skin,
he wanted simply to grow old here,
to grow wiser, to breathe new and more music,
to make good art in the place he loved the most,
one humble branch in the tree of life.

Now the tour buses bring daily to these Strawberry Fields
legions from all the lands,
murmuring in all of the languages,
cameras flashing, flowers strewn,
prayers offered up in singularly profound sincerity and respect,
still seeking clarity on the vision
that John, artist of the soul,
perhaps the first citizen of the world,
held up for us to yearn for, to seek after,
not that long ago.

(8)

It is a seventeen step rise to the hallowed entry of St. Patrick's Cathedral;
the grandiose brass doors are made to mimic the gates of the Holy City,
made to whisper the power of Rome.
When these gates first opened
the church's spire pointing to heaven
constituted the very highest manmade point in Manhattan.
These gates include the bronzed suprahuman heights
of six medieval saints, standing guard;
they are polished weekly by Miguel, a native of Guatemala,
the diocesan coins for this chore forwarded home
to mother and siblings who worship in a cathedral
with a mud floor and tin roof
where they chant for peace and know more well than the archdiocesan Cardinal,
steaming vichyssoise awaiting the conclusion of his homily,
that more food would help bring more peace.

It was upon this dias that at nineteen
as I wept before an RCA television in Ann Arbor
that Robert Kennedy's memory was canonized by the last of the brothers.
Some men dream of things that never were.
Now the mass is being officiated over by an arch-bishop.
His golden embroidered frock and aged, tenored, withered voice

incants words of righteousness, ritual,
honoring forgiveness, peace, and understanding.

Elsewhere in the city the same scene is acted out
by esteemed leaders of an array of ancient traditions
a Marquis de Sade patchwork of liturgical propositions,
in places like the Collegiate Church on Lexington,
dating to General Washington and the Revolution,
and Riverside Church in Morningside,
with its lineage dating to founder John D. Rockefeller,
simultaneously ravager of Holy Land oil,
richest man in the world,
born again Christian, and consummate philanthropist,
with Dr. James A. Forbes preaching his vast brains out,
coming on down now,
trying to assimilate these archaic methodologies,
or at the Congregation Rodelph Sholom on 83rd St.,
as well as the other 620 synagogues in this town,
or at the Mosque Majid-Al Ameen on 23rd St.

Fortunately most of the butt shined pews stand empty
occupied only by scattered largely half-asleep robots and the elderly
destined like this manner of worship not to be here for long.
Islam, Chistendom, and Jewry trudging onward,
sustained by one common God?
Sustained like arid weeds between the cracks in
the blacktop of abandoned parking lots.

My own blood boils as it will
with my own brand of highly purified first press righteous indignation.
With each prayer offered up, each cup raised, each verse recited,
the futility of this mass self-assurance of rightness
the misguided goodness gone to waste
drives me insane

as I sit on my park bench and study the Times,
peer at CNN,
watch the planes cruise above,
feel the harsh aroma of scorched earth and bodies emanating
throughout the atmosphere as across the whole of this earth,
innocent children die in the name of this religious primalism.
I have come to know these rituals, all of them.
The time has come for a mass burial, a final ceasefire,
a final leap into the awareness that we can all love each other,
regardless of the obvious color differentials,
the stew of ethnic differences,
the passion of deeply held religious pieties,
ironically religion the final sin.

I see the roadmap in children at play
who do not seem to notice their array of skin tones;
toddler colleagues, the future
oblivious to the array of languages and dialects,
accepting each other as equals, oblivious to the differences.

It is finally their future and they will be able
to engage it if we do not deprive them of the opportunity.

Is it that difficult to see that the sanctity of human life,
the power of god coursing through the arteries of every living person,
that therein lies God,
not in these ancient religion museums,
these limping canonical armories that hold us to the past.

I feel the presence of a post-denominational spirituality rising,
upon which the foundation of the future peace will be given its birth.

(9)

November 1, 2004

Joe Bushkin died today at the age of 87.
He was born in a brownstone at the corner of 103rd and Park Avenue in 1916.
His father, a barber from the Ukraine, played cello between haircuts.
Joe himself played with Billie Holiday and Frank Sinatra and Benny Goodman and
Bunny Berigan,
served in the Air Force and lived a life devoted to Swing.
He is survived by his wife and four daughters,
of New York, San Francisco, and Santa Barbara.

Is this a great country?

(10)

November 3.

Today the President is smirking,
perhaps his most outstanding single ability.
He looks silly
like a gloating second string hick B high school quarterback
who just accidentally won the big game
despite a predilection for running into the wrong end zone.

In the City this gloat seems both pathetic and absurd.

Does this bloodthirsty band of conservative morons,
this self-aggrandizing slime wad of bigoted, sexist, homophobic dirtballs,
this shitpile of shrunken dick racist hate mongers,
this new American theocracy,
really believe that buying the minds of a brain dead electorate
can alter the inevitability
that in the long run it is Truth that will prevail,
and that in truth the genuine promise of history
is that the intrinsic goodness of mankind will endure and survive
as its power dwarfs the petty smallness of the pipsqueak turd in the White House?

(11)

"By hard, honest labor I've dug all the large words out of my vocabulary.
I never write "metropolis",
because I can get the same money for "city"."

Mark Twain
Speech to the Associated Press, New York City
1906

(12)

The Marathon

It is evening.
I stand at the finish line.
The bleachers are empty.
Only a few straggling workers making preparations
and a few twitchy runners who can't wait
taking their last preparatory laps.

In the morning there will be a race
and highly conditioned runners from across the globe
will cross this line in search of fame, glory,
or some new knowledge of themselves otherwise unattainable.

Their faces will be etched with varying degrees of pain.

Theirs will be a depth of fatigue that I have known before.
The spasm of the overstretched tendons,
the hollow aching of the pleura,
the haunting of regrets for the undone,
are not foreign to my own being.

Pain in the legs, exhaustion in the lungs,
a fullness in the heart which I remember well.
The feeling of having done a lot,
but not having done enough,
which I am destined to take with me.

I feel fortunate that
it is their race to run now.
I am glad to observe,
and pass the torch to this progeny of seekers ready for the run.

My mind turns to my own band of children and the utter trust
I have in their capacity to carry this forward,
the immensity of the talents they still are growing into,
the willingness of their spirits.
I stand both humble and sober before the human capacity for wrong,
but am much more amazed by the general rightness of things.

I am tired but honestly have more energy left than I expected to have.

The truth which I have been in search of,
which I thought would arrive in flashing crimson flames,
or in a perfectly turned choice of words,
or gasping at the view from some pinnacle or precipice,
or zigzagging across some field of broken glass staggering toward a goal line,
has arrived in a manner
more akin to the slow drip by drip melting of a block of ice,
the miracle of nature opening itself to welcome a new spring,
the freshness of a new beginning arising as a phoenix
from past struggles which were not as impossible as they seemed at the time.

It is the fairest of the seasons;
and even though the little hand continues to gallop along,
the big hand has settled into a graceful canter,
and an even bigger hand seems to hold me with kindness,
and ease me gently along.

(13)

Bob Dylan

It's not dark yet, but it's getting there.

(14)

December 4.

It is midnight.
Advent has tiptoed in upon us.
The late hour is belied
by the ongoing fluorescent glow
from the billion Con Edison tweaking lights of Times Square;
ET phone home;

the streets remain crowded with the exiting theater goers,
their faces still painted with the tear, or the awe, or the shock, or the hilarity,
of the evening's repast.

We stroll arm in arm,
our own hearts warmed to the unhurried Midtown magic,
Christmas bells, stray Santas, scarved skaters, Americans posing for snapshots;
we turn the corner and approach arm in arm to the foot of the Tree.

Our tree.
Our village tree, our people's tree, our country's tree,
all of which we have long believed in.

It is in fact a miracle,
with each of the infinite array of glittering lights
matching a counter universe of glow in our common heart.

Thus the miracle, the truth, the final wisdom.

It is all about the love.

The pursuit of love.
The relentless pursuit.
The thrilling pursuit.
The painful gut-wrenching pursuit.
The ecstatic pursuit.
The brain emptying pursuit.
The tearful heartbreaking pursuit.
The unending pursuit.

Here in the heart of this great City,
here at the foot of this great tree,
here in the eye of our own storm,

here anonymously amid the passing festive throngs,
miraculously,
we have arrived here together,
souls meshed for the long journey,
on the eve of this coming season of peace among men,
with peace in our hearts,
and a bursting love for each other.

7

HUMAN SEXUALITY

WHEN YOU PUT a Boy and a Girl

The little kept secret in creative writing whether fiction, biography, expository, commercial, reportorial, journalistic, in order to garnish full attention of a vast readership, the key is of course to include plenty of sex. Just ask the writer who composed the tome about shades of grey, which I always thought was just what made great black and white photography elegant and ambiguous. Who knew? Haven't read it but certainly she got paid better than we do for looking at a bunch of sore throats though I'm sure there were some seriously sore throats before her book was over. Anyway this chapter is my attempt to capture that audience. Enjoy. Probably won't be much heavy breathing.

I could of course deal with this by composing a chronology of the epic unending historically epochal cavalcade of sexual seduction and conquest which I personally have modestly achieved over my own decades, all within the context of the romantic adventure of the 44 years of my physically and spiritually intriguing marriage, but I am way too private for that. Easier to rat out my patients.

By way of both introduction and summary it can be stated in an inclusive way that there is likely little in the known universe more confoundingly complex than the roots, development, and execution of the drama of the sexual nature of homo sapiens, monsieurs and madame in equal proportion. If I ever thought that this was a subject that could be grasped adequately enough to be of effective clinical service, that idea has been long disavowed. I have also long ago rejected the notion of ever achieving that status. Just when you think you have heard or seen it all, a new twist is encountered. Take 549. Cameras, action.

When trying to measure the power wielded by the sexual within, just think of a few presidential candidates with the big prize in sight unable to resist for a roll in the hay with a bimbo, not to mention a long string of occupants of the oval office willing to risk their facade of integrity for an occasional quickie, or a professional golfer making a billion a year so attracted to cocktail waitresses that Nike can go to hell, or Latin emperors, Russian Czars, Chinese Dynasty Mavens. Never mind the Ordinated elite. You get the point. As I think about it my professional colleagues over the years have tended toward the sexual kosher in their private lives, as far as I know. As I think about it further being the father confessor and captain of the seas of biology gone amuck might tend to have a eunuchfication effect. Spellcheck that word if you dare. Though an occasional exception comes to mind.

As I think about it further, though, I am not sure that the great unwashed masses don't tend more toward the Chauncey Gardner philosophy, "I like to watch."

Anyway.

One Saturday back in Lenox the floor to ceiling screen door at the rear end of our stretched out side porch, circa 1800, really needed re-screening and I devoted an eight hour Spring Saturday to disemboweling it, replacing the old with the new, fixing it down one tack at a time and restoring it to its seven foot tall rightful place. I was assisted in this by three of my four daughters, the fourth still un-conceived, and our faithful dog Jackson, magnificent Black Beauty of a creature, half Labrador, half Shepard, epitome of consummate canine masculinity. Only to say that at 4:45 just as I was preparing to light the charcoal, Jackson escalated a full trot from the kitchen through the family room like a Kentucky Derby thoroughbred heading around the far turn and crashed through the tightly locked freshly appointed screen door like a knife cutting through soft butter. Some poignant fragrance in the air creating a fixation in

Jackson of doing some consummating of his own. Loved that dog. I have witnessed a lot of other no matter whats. But that one was an excellent lesson in never underestimating the force of love unrequited. To this day you still see a lot of dogs roaming the streets of Lenox village that look a little like Jackson.

I have made it my business to get a feel for this aspect of ourselves in an historic sense; few problems cannot be better induced through a good long term fund of factual information and a broad context. In fact an interest and some knowledge of biological evolution, human anthropology specifically, mixed with a solid understanding of the basic medical sciences are of necessity in analyzing a wide variety of medical problems.

My pursuit of such understanding led me to studying the human family tree from its origins. I have had ready access to the American Museum of Natural History where I have spent long hours wandering, wondering, studying. The Hall of Human Origins I find is as fascinating of a way of spending a few Saturday afternoon hours as any hobbyist could concoct. Engrossing. So reading and viewing, following out our early lines and migrations etc. brought me to an admiration for the Neanderthal family, one might say of man, though it is taught that the Neanderthals, who did enjoy a much longer run of civilized existence in western Europe than it looks like Homo Sapiens is likely to manage, and did in fact develop a social system which flowed well and with great longevity, did ultimately come to its end in a biological blind alley, their line coming to a final demise, only to be wondered at. Though in the office I do occasionally have the sense of interviewing a true unmitigated Neanderthal.

This in contrast to various predecessors of our own lineage who stumbled over many of the organizational challenges at which the Neanderthals succeeded. My attempt to get this sequence of events ordered in my head became more confused when studying new information from DNA research indicating that DNA recombinant from Neanderthals does show up in modern man here and there. I brought this quandary up to my dear friend Dr. Albert Harper, anthropologist, famous crime scene analyst, doctor of law, elite medical examiner, general all around academic encyclopedia. Expecting an esoteric explanation which I hoped to be able to handle the depth of, he responded with something like, "Well the general anthropological principle here is that when you put a boy and a girl alone in a room together, they will fuck." Probably true. Even though this was a new insight to me it did bring together a level of logic and understanding which previously I had found highly elusive in dealing with this facet of my patients' lives clinically.

Let's start with Donald and Marge. It is difficult to think on one without the other in that their mother-son relationship was of the Bobsey twin mold which a family practitioner encounters daily.

We see sisters who are not twins but might as well be. Either that or the doctor has contracted acute double vision. Husband and wife combos attached at the waste - quite often this attachment occurs when the gentlemen retires and finds the life of a faithful puppy dog to be the pot of gold at the end of the rainbow. Mom and daughter with overlapping personalities are a dime a dozen. The many situations where a child at an age formerly viewed as senior citizen moving in to save the life of an increasingly fragile aging parent, guiding the loved one to a gentle passing can be most endearing to watch as a life of mutual love and respect is faithfully fulfilled. The pushing upward of our life expectancy has increased the frequency of that dynamic out of necessity but it remains edifying to be in support of, some form of old world virtue managing to survive in the present. You also find the supportive friend, neighbor, grandchild, cousin who find the time and energy to be there for someone in a time of prolonged need, also admirable if at times difficult to explain. Some of those giving individuals are at the same end of a chain of similarly constructed relationships repetitively, i.e. having codependent flair. It often occurs that some of these individuals would have made excellent doctors or nurses if they weren't so pure of heart and sound of mind.

Donald and Marge were inseparable though my first encounter was entering an exam room and meeting Donald by himself, straight as an arrow, pleasantly friendly with a mildly reserved smile, nerdish in a major way with well pressed starched shirt sans button down or any other accoutrement, hair cropped tightly with an emphasis on neatness but assiduously avoiding any sense of style. A well-crafted dork. He had this tightened twist of the mouth smile in response to anything ironic that always reminded me of a senior church lady sharing gossip at the card table with close hen friends. His body mechanics were a match to this demeanor, an old lady in a young man's body. I am certain that Marge was only a few feet away in the waiting room, probably with binoculars and a periscope. Maybe a stethoscope to the thin wall.

"What can I do for you?" Donald's response was a cut to the chase question answering a question. "Well I was wondering if it can be normal to have absolutely no sex drive." Hmmm. We went through a bit more exhaustive series of questions aimed at meting out the possibility of some endocrinologic issues, getting to know him more personally - the setting of his life story and significant relationships, etc. - the markers of his life, past medical history (none), and a fairly complete physical exam with special attention to hormonally influenced areas - muscle mass, hair growth and distribution, gonadal anatomic features. This was followed by a comprehensive lab investigation of general health parameters as well as obtaining some hormone levels, testosterone, thyroid, cortisol, all of which were to prove normal. He stuck to his story that he had no sexual urges of any sort, not toward women, not toward men, not toward children, not toward photographic images, not towards the neighbor's dog.

We left it at that - I was direct that I really didn't know the cause of his non-libidinous worldview but I did confirm that it was at the least highly unusual and definitely important and that the matter should probably be explored further with a caring and competent therapist. He indicated that he would discuss it "with Mother". The subject did not come up again over the next decade or so. I would see him occasionally for a physical or some minor medical issue, always accompanied by "Mother".

Their daily routine was to rise at a nice early Protestant hour each morning and have their Cornflakes together while packing their brown bag lunches for later on at their adjacent sit down technical jobs at "The GE", before completing their shifts and walking together to the parking lot and heading to one or the other local family style restaurants to select some spaghetti or a burger or on the frisky occasion the hot roast beef sandwich and share animatedly the high point of their day's activities at the GE before home, to straighten out a closet or a cupboard, polishing a spoon or a vase, donning the older cardigan and comfy slippers for a TV show or two before an early hour time for jammies and nighty-nighty in what I always hoped were separate bedrooms.

Parenthetically, whenever I ever asked either of them about Donald's father, their response was an identical, precise and succinct, "Oh, he drank" as if that more than explained. Really .It probably did. Why she might need a different spouse? Why he might need one reliable parent?

Marge became the more regular patient. She was also neatly well-kept, polite and demure at all times, not unaware of the outside world but not in the least interested in what went on there. Her clothes were clean and also they were clean. Very clean. She shared her son's coy sense of humor, or vice-versa. Her hair was always fixed in the same perma-frost permanent - silvery and stiffly curled - certainly renewed weekly. What did Donald do for that endless hour when she was being coiffed by the beautician? He almost certainly had read all of that waiting room's Ladies Home Journals twice. She was bright, not inarticulate, though a bit of a hypochondriac and rather unappreciative of the art of brevity in the description of bodily symptoms, especially when involving something fascinating like some dramatic change in her stool size, frequency, or configuration. And I don't mean her stool at the GE. They would occasionally make reference to their Sunday attendance at the local First Baptist Church, the services of which I knew they would never arrive at without steadfast, reverent, ardent punctuality.

This went on for a long number of years. The coziness, the intimacy, the regularities in all matters and things, the mopping and tidying up on Saturday mornings before off to the grocery, the naughtiness of chuckling over Seinfeld on Sunday evenings, the security provided by two good GE jobs with full union benefits (?remember those) all seemed to work well for both of them.

Then things changed. At a youngish 58 even though she had always been in some way born old, Marge developed an aggressive ovarian cancer and within weeks absented this previously heavily controlled and measured out scene. Donald was 38 and alone in the world. The applecart went kappooofff.

Donald not long thereafter required a fairly long acute care psychiatric admission on our local psych unit, Two Jones. It was about time he had some Jones in his life actually. He became unwound. When I visited him on the locked unit he was neat and clean though not quite to his former standards, friendly and cooperative but clearly also suffering from a broken heart. Shaky. He eventually recovered enough to return to the loneliness of his home and his job at the GE but that chapter in fact proved to be over as he would repetitively unravel, end up back on 2J for some re-balancing and never was able to regain his footing in the work environment. In his early forties he was judged psychiatrically disabled and since that time, now a couple of more decades, has been receiving his weekly benefits from Mother/Father GE or one its insurance subsidiaries.

I didn't see or hear from him for about five years.

He then re-presented as if our relationship had been uninterrupted looking for some help in getting restarted, admitting that he had been quite depressed "for a while" but wanting to get unstuck.

We started from scratch. "Well, what have you got going on?" A full and fresh update on his physical health which I did not find beyond repair. Though he had lost a chunk of weight. And many long discussions on how one might go about putting together a personal life. What kind of activities do you take an interest in? How can a person make a few friends? What has happened in clothes over the last 25 years. And such. We also started an anti-depressant. A psychiatrist might identify this as a period of medical office based re-parenting.

He would return every month or so with baited breath, report in detail on his small victories and occasional defeats. With each visit his clothes became a bit swifter, his body mechanics a bit more loosely jointed, his hair a longer cut. He did always look as if someone else had dressed him. After a while I gave him a leash of a couple of months upon which he returned with apparel appropriate for competing in the Tour de France, his muscles, once pale and flaccid, now toned and tanned. Donald? He related that his shiny new $2,000 Italian racing bike was parked out front.

I didn't see him for a couple of years and figured he was probable okay.

He then reappeared for a scheduled visit and after pleasantries indicated that he wanted to reinvestigate the sexual question which we had opened with two decades before. We talked about dating, internet dating sites, where to go to meet what type of individual, how to dress, how to make conversation. My own teenagers I don't think ever needed that particular talk. Nevertheless he would return every month or two for update and coaching, each time with good progress. After a few such months I entered the room to find him fashionably put together, now a little hair overhang on his forehead locks, smiling, engaging, a little affected but not without some cool. He announced that he was in a relationship, that it was going great, and that he was most unequivocally gay and not minding it at all. All of the above has been having a happy ending for the last twenty years.

I learned a lot from this.

There is the obvious that in our lives we as human beings sacrifice immeasurable losses of the full fulfillment of what we can be on the altar of family dynamic dictated constraints and historically predetermined social morays and biases.

I also learned that sexuality is a powerfully innate part of all of us, the healthy fulfillment of which has a far prettier outcome than the oppression of basic, innate parts of what we are.

Are we getting sexy enough yet?

It occurs to me that treating sexually transmitted disease has never been a big item in our practice, though a college campus based physician would have to get pretty good at it. On the other hand we do get called on once in a while to discretely check for the same following a recent indiscretion or suspected partner's indiscretion. This interaction is often charged with a moderate level of panic or some hopped up rage, neither of which tends to be dissipated by reassurance that most of the conditions we look for are pretty treatable. Color the patient's faces at these visits a guilty pale pastel.

The phenomenon of an internationally traveling high level business executive returning from various on the other side of the world countries in a diaphoretic state of feverish fear and guilt. They usually say, "Doc, I can't believe I would do something like this!" I couldn't generally agree more, except you do have a boy and a girl issue. I try to assuage their guilt and relieve their state of agitated fearfulness without endorsing the behavior or validating the insanity in any way.

When I first entered practice Herpes Genitalis was not a condition lacking serious or widespread dissemination. The slogan "Herpes is Forever" pervaded the media and the nation's license plates. The advent of antiviral antibiotics, both safe and effective have removed the sting of that onus. Most of the people who still have outbreaks have them rarely and know how to treat them on their own. The ubiquitous condomization of below the belt interpersonal communication has also helped immensely.

When I first started HIV disease was something rumored to be a problem in Haiti. Within a few years a terrible epidemic had ensued on our own shores, no hamlets left unaffected. We saw enough Aids patients to satisfy our intellectual curiosity though a physician practicing in Provincetown or Greenwich Village would have to make this disease a central focus in their professional concerns and expertise. Fortunately, modern pharmacologic therapy and the condom have also come to the rescue in this area and now HIV is a back burner issue. Merciful God.

Probably the most frequent complaint in the sexual sphere is what we refer to as "E.D." or erectile dysfunction. I have also witnessed considerable evolution over the years relative to this touchy issue, no pun intended. Interesting that I don't recall any mention of the problem in medical school even in cursory fashion. My own assumption on male sexual performance through the years was that all men basically were interested in having sex whenever the occasion arose (no pun intended) and were able to perform fine and dandy until old age set in, maybe at 38 or so, when things would gradually peter out (sorry, no pun intended). Then along came Viagra. I soon came to realize that tons of men were underperformers and much too embarrassed to bring it up (no pun intended) especially since there was nothing to do except bemoan this limping to the finish line, (no pun intended).

Also interesting that now a decade into the new and definitely better era men in general who find themselves in need are so much more casual in bringing up the matter (I'll stop now, too easy) and enlisting assistance. The furtive whispering and clandestine calling of a pharmacy 62 miles away and all have been dismissed to so what. From the get-go it has seemed to me that it was a very exact 50% of the time that the request for a prescription like on TV was generated by the guy's wife. As opposed to the 100% of the time when upon turning to leave the room after doing a 45 minute exam and the patient said, "Oh, by the way,…" that it turned out to be some question about Viagra that maybe some friend was wondering about.

Also interesting how social tendencies around the state of undressing have evolved. Each generation seems a bit more relaxed about their bodies and maybe in a couple of more centuries we will catch up with the south of France. I once take care of a group three Catholic nuns (is that a redundancy?) and believe me the complexity of layered dress attendant with that profession in the old days was mindboggling. Try breaking into Fort Knox, definitely easier than memorizing the nine overlapping layers to the human abdominal wall which they could easily stretch to twenty-two.

My own stance on dealing with the need to have patients trust you in evaluation of any and all body parts have never been a matter to be taken lightly. I don't particularly like to be poked at myself. I believe that both genders, all ages, all ethnicities, all IQ levels, etc. does not alter the fundamental need to continuously deserve the trust that people place in you. Examining men of course is not much different than sharing the YMCA locker room facilities. Most of the conversation while business is conducted is about the Red Sox anyway. A little more sensitive for a male physician with a female patient but not that much as it seems like the vast majority of all ages get that the physical function of the body is what we are trained to deal with. In addition I do have a wife and four daughters about whose privacy and integrity I have serious respect for and can only treat all women in the same fashion I would prefer for my family. I do have testosterone floating around in my bloodstream but I have never felt anything feeling remotely sexual in dealing with patients. My awareness of the awkwardness being experienced by the receiver of our attempt to help totally over trumps and wanting to minimize that is the priority. I suppose all of that goes without saying but I reiterate, transgression of inviolable physical and emotional boundaries between doctor and patient constitute a potential minefield I have never wanted anything to do with.

Ethical self-righteousness aside I would submit this recollection to substantiate my point. I am working at the Family Health Center one busy morning about fifteen years again when Cindy called from the set of The Morning After Hollywood movie where she was employed tutoring a child actor, Julia. She wondered whether I would be able to spend some time with Meryl Streep who played the part of a pediatrician in the movie and needed some hospital procedural modeling. I told her that I was swamped but send her over and I would arrange for something. Cindy was a little shocked that evening when I told her that I had the hospital anesthesiologist deal with Meryl. In hindsight I am sure that Meryl would have been quite taken with me but shoot as lovely of a lady as she is, she never was and still isn't even in the same league with my wife. Love you, Cin. You're the best honey.

Then there is of course the mundane of men and women in general, mostly husbands and wives but in this day and age spanning enumerable types of relationships with varying level and types of commitments, developing bedroom problems. One thing which I have learned across the eons is that despite the wonderful ways in which men and women are different, including how we compose a matching set of jumper cables capable of procreation, once you get past the external differences and some of the infrastructure, men and women are more like each other than not. We all require acknowledgement, we need to be seen, recognized, shown affection, given respect, have our basic needs of food, shelter, protection from the elements, as well as the basic needs of conversation, intimacy, sharing, kindness, given and taken.

There is major overlap in a doctor's office between matters sexual and how things are going in the relationship as a whole. There is the obvious that women are in fact more relationship driven and sexually reactive to things like tenderness, loyalty, compliments, consideration, whereas men are more superficially physical in arousal and attack. Clichéd truth but truth. Thus the TV network and the team ownership get more male customers watching when they put aerobic and plastic surgery embossed professional model cheerleader types on the field and more female customers when they have interviews post game with modest, sincere, boyish athletes who begin their interview by thanking God, blowing tearful kisses to their wife and four children back home in Georgia, and not forgetting aw shucks to thank their Sunday school teacher at the corner church.

This plays out in marriages in trouble in that the wife usually describes various forms of maltreatment - physical (the doctor needs to point out against the law), financial, verbal (pet names like bitch and worse), which the doctor may be the only person in a position to help the poor lady with - hello, this is being abuse, as these individuals usually have self- images beaten down to shreds. The fact that any sexual attraction could survive such onslaught is preposterous, though it does behoove the doctor to keep in mind that there are occasional individuals who for bizarre deeply-situated reasons tend to provoke and thrive on mistreatment.

The male version is more likely to refer to a lack of sex, often preceded by disclaimers like, "Well I told her we would have more sex if she would lose some of her fat ass." Where do you start? Talk about re-parenting. "How can you feel like sex when all she does is complain about my new truck, how much I go fishing, my very best friend sleeping on the floor in our family room, the fact that I went to a perfectly innocent bachelor party for my old buddy at a strip club, that I only want sex after two or three six-packs, etc.

The fundamental issue here is that the responsibilities of raising young children has created a population of women grown up and responsible enough to carry on adult relationships and too many who expect to be pampered and juvenilized in adulthood as they were in childhood from the time they put on their first Little League uniform.

With humor, some male bonding, some stern fathering, some basic what you should have learned in Kindergarten, a lot of these guys can be helped. Nothing wrong with saving a marriage here and there. A lot of male sexist behavior is uglier on the surface than truly intended. They say never blame on malice that which can be explained by sheer stupidity.

All of which begs the question relevant I suppose to anthropologists, sociologists, as well as physicians, perhaps all of us: Why the vast difference in sexual appetite individual to individual human being. I have found that there are many married couples with a shared indifference to sexual activity, often at strikingly young ages and they tend to do fine. Likewise I have come across seemingly equal in frequency situations where both ends of the partnership stay ready and willing with great regularity, often into quite advanced years, also a compatible arrangement. Problems are obviously more likely to arise when one partner or the other starts out or becomes less interested which can be stressful or fatal to an otherwise good relationship or provoke a variety of acting out behaviors doing no one any good. I know that many sexual liberals view the conservative outlook in this area unenlightened. My experience is that many of those enlightened individuals end up getting treated for a lot of STD's, paying a lot of alimony, losing important relationships in their lives (their children, former in-laws of many years), and using a ton of Viagra trying to maintain their false sense of virility. Sad.

A word about geriatric sexuality: it exists. Got a large charge one time when chatting very personally with an 88 year old and still cute lady who probably could have gotten away stretching the truth about her age. She had kept me informed as she ushered into her life a new boyfriend quite a few years after the loss of her husband to cancer after many years of happy marriage. As the wise doctor congratulated her on her pro-life openness and pointed out to her that it was great to have some companionship even at an age where the physical was no longer important she responded with overt candor, "Oh but doctor, I love the sex!!"

I have a lot to say about the phenomenon of sexual addiction but we'll get to that where it belongs when we address addictive illness, another fascinating chapter yet to come.

So why do we all have this enormous drive - to reproduce, to be raptured, to be gratified - over and again for as long as we live.

I don't know for sure.

I suppose the answer is somewhere in the same realm with why the maple tree outside my window here in a few weeks is going to blossom and shed about four billion helicopter seeds across my yard. There are approximately 200,000,000 mostly viable spermatozoa in each ejaculate. At birth the female human infant's ovaries are blessed with around 50,000 potential ova. Go figure.

What I do know that is at the best the sexual within us constitutes when properly honored and executed the best of what we can experience in the psychospiritual realm of this earthly experience. Love between two human beings in its purest for in my most humble opinion is the closest we can come as mortal creatures to being touched by the hand of God. Worth working for, worth trying to be a better person for, worth any struggle, any sacrifice.

Thank you God for this very special fountain of joy.

Or as Yogi Berra famously said, "90% of it is half mental." I always figured that while Mickey Mantle and Whitey Ford were too tanked to finish off anything glorious with the barfly of the night,

Yogi was at home having a great time in bed and at the breakfast table with the girl he would stay married to for sixty years.

GRAND DESIGN

It's only life, after all.
> The Indigo Girls

Oh ultimate architect, master chemist,
> transcendent electrician, sculptor extraordinaire,
> I stand in awe.

From the perspective of my own lengthening view,
> my final exam coming into sight, ne imminent,
> disembarkation inevitable.

I stand in awe.

That you reduce so deftly infinity into the elemental,
> that you expand the ordinary to the power maximus,
> that humility, that humor, that rapture
> so easily coalesce in your hand.

Forward entropy, reverse entropy become the same.

I remember the touch of handfuls of warm sand
> arid from the scorch of summer sun
> falling between my fingers as I repose
> mass reduced to steady march of identical members
> equal particles of silicon dioxide reacted upon
> without judgment by gravity,
> sands of time,

each performing a ballet of its own to the earth center
each grain for me to incorporate, file, enjoin, recall,
sensory ganglia, long tracts, parietal neurons lit, rearranged,
laughing children dancing in their circles about me.

I remember the translucence of water
    broken by the grainy shellacked paddle surface,
    wood harvested from nearby forest tract
    now pared to tool,
    violating the surface of the glassy liquid silence
    pure mountain lake aqueous essence
    sliced into its billion diaphanous parts
    set on reverse course
    flowing wave passing in its own paced freedom,
    illuminated for that microsecond into uncountable reams of color,
    solar effect on prismed dihydrogen oxide molecules mechanically disrupted
    by that astrally reincarnated Iroquois,
    and puerile princess, heiress to this largesse
    breathing in tandem the same ticks of time.

I remember it all.

And I envision the openness of the night's sky
    seen from beyond our atmospheric boundaries
    out above our gravity
    out among the intergalactic
    I envision
    a Milky Way of artist stars
    each glowing with its own luminescence
    each the transfiguration of an artist's earthly candle
    soul lights burning, creating still
    those who have spoken to me in this time.

I see these star cells connected and intermingled
    by strands of celestial beams,

energy forms, bent light, cosmic photons -
an AT+T switchboard diagram of the universe
based on the afterglow of collective creativities,
design my own.

The poet, the painter, the composer, the thespian,
      all acting upon the giant theater of the universe.

Duke Ellington is aboard the A train.

Yo Yo Ma wands cello strings stretched like energy fields
      pole to pole the length of the Silk Road.

Walt Whitman stands atop the balustrade of the Brooklyn Bridge
      and heralds his city below
      "Multitudes! Yes! Multitudes!"

Beckett grunts and moans and moroses and writhes
      in the ecstatic rapture of his own agony.

John Lennon sits with legs crossed
      and recites the lines to Imagine
      as the Buddha sit and nods approval
      while Jesus (too much wine) does a whimsical soft-shoe at their side.

Caruso sings to Vesuvius,
      Shakespeare does the Times Sunday Crossword (backwards in Greek),
      Virgil spots his distant shore,
      Louis triumphantly trumpets the Saints for the saints.

Dickens and Bellow play a hand of gin,
      O'Neil and Hemingway tip a glass of gin,
      Hendrix plays the anthem on nuclear rays (with his toes),
      while Springsteen is being reborn to run.

John Coltrane blows hot,
> while Miles blows cool,
> and Thelonius and Johann Sebastian share the bench
> to knock off some ragtime fortissimo.

Bo Jangles be a tappin' his toes.
> loving the sight of Fred and Ginger waltzing across space,
> Gershwin tickling out Rhapsody in Blue solo.

What do they most want to say to each other?

Is this the peace that is to come?

I laugh.

And am happy.

And certain.

This is my dream.

And I offer it up with reverence
> along with
> the bits added on by the lines
> that happened to cross in me
> and I pass it forward
> to this masterwork of children now to speak for me
> and defer gratefully to all of my kind
> to carry on.

Recognizing, the grandness of it all in this late moment,
      of the ultimate permanence of these equations,
      their delicate immutability, their velvety steadiness,
      that the consciousness granted to us is without weight,
      it had no beginning and will have no end,
      that it will continue on,
      like this always flowing river of being,
      that has always been,
      and always will be.

8

CARDIOVASCULAR HEALTH

TICK TOCK TICK Tock

It is lovely September in the Berkshires, the time of the year when a sunny after-noon can ignite a panoply of foliage chromaticity - reds, gold, oranges - that can be painted across a deeply blue sky canvas in a way that can make your heart want to stop, though that may be a less than apt metaphor when you are intern on a cardiol-ogy rotation as I was in the autumn of 1972. It was on one such glorious afternoon that I was called to the Emergency Unit of St. Luke's Hospital to evaluate a young man whom everyone just referred to as Anthony, partly because he appeared with a level of frequency in the same unit with the same complaint, pain in the left anterior part of his chest, and partly because he had lived in the prevailingly Italian neighbor-hood his entire life, a neighborhood where everyone knew everyone, and their hard to count cousins as well.

Anthony's electrocardiogram was non -ischemic in any acute way which was usually the case with him though there was evidence of an old myocardial infarction. He was only 32 but had had his previous MI at the tender age of 28 four years previ-ously. On the phone, his attending pointed out to me that he tended to be a cardiac neurotic (obsessed with every twinge in his body as a possible heart attack) but that given his history we agreed that he should be admitted for observation.

That meant having daily EKG's and serial cardiac enzymes done on his blood looking for evidence of cardiac insult which we carried out in customary protocol for a few days, during which time I had a chance to get to know him and appreciate his easy-going manner. I learned from him a lot about the nature of growing up Italian in Pittsfield, the closely-knit nature of the community, the shared family values which included a pretty much pre-ordained life plan which included definite first communion at Mt. Carmel Church, one day graduating from St. Joseph's High School, marrying your sweetheart named Angela or whom you met in kindergarten and went to the senior prom with, and probably working at a well-paying job a mile away at the General Electric Power Transformer factory, and definitely eating a lot of spaghetti along the way.

Anthony was of this vintage and had the genuinely good looks of the same with deeply tanned Sicilian features including a thick head of luxuriant black hair, think Frankie Avalon with a New England accent. I am certain that his wife had him picked out by third grade. Anthony was fully relaxed on the medical floor when not having chest pain and wandered freely with his pajama sleeves folded up nattily, chatting with the nurses and aides and orderlies and custodians all of whom knew and liked him. He would spend a good part of his time lounging on the long screened in porch which stretched the length of the old brick hospital, appointed with garden type furniture for patients and families to enjoy. Usually he would have a few cigarettes while taking his leisure, perhaps sharing a couple with an old friend or two.

On the third hospital day I was summonsed to evaluate Anthony for another episode of chest pain which could certainly pass as angina and on this occasion was associated with a level of diaphoresis, a distinctive cold sweat. The EKG still showed nothing but we transferred him to the coronary unit, which was basically several old hospital rooms with walls removed to allow for a string of cubicles where patients could be placed on monitors which a specially trained nurse could sit and watch as every heartbeat was recorded. Anthony kept having frequent runs of chest heaviness which came to be only relieved by intravenous morphine. Some of the staff thought that he was enjoying the morphine too much. In contradistinction to that theory it was at one a.m. that I was called to the unit for a Mayday situation as Anthony was in full cardiac arrest. All attempts at resuscitation were met with failure. As was customary I placed a call to his private physician to inform him of the events. I remember being concerned that the attending sounded so soundly asleep that he might have a difficult time relating over the phone the heart-breaking information that she was now a widow and their two children had lost their father.

The nurse attending the situation mentioned to me as a patient in the office about twenty years later that I had commented at the time on how difficult it must be to convey report of such a tragic event and perhaps the family should have been called to the hospital to have that conversation.

Move the clock forward a bit. It is Superbowl Sunday 2010 and I am enjoying the football game and some chicken wings with a few old friends as one of my friends relates with only a little bemusement the unusual events of his previous week. Lonnie is a long term Pittsfield family lawyer well liked in the community and very hard-working. Apparently after getting to work on Monday morning he started to have a funny feeling in his chest which passed as he went about his work. Then after a while it returned and he indicated to his secretary that maybe she should take him down to the ER to get checked. He did that and in less than an hour was on his was to Baystate Medical Center in Springfield for a cardiac catheterization which was performed that afternoon, identifying two occluding arteries which were rapidly bypassed with teflon coated stents. He rested overnight and was discharged home in the morning to be driven home by his wife where he rested for the remainder of the day and then returned to work on Wednesday morning.

As instructed he started on a few medications and made an appointment to see his own local doctor in a few days and to go back to Springfield for follow-up in a month or so. We all enjoyed the party especially the delicious deep fried chicken wings and even more so the elated fans of the New York Giants who were in attendance. The Patriots fans left a little forlorn.

How has this amazing transformation in expected clinical outcome come about?

Basically through a mountain of very hard work.

There is an army of physicians dedicated to clinical research which stretches the world around, funded largely through public means, grants from our federal government and similarly throughout other modern nations. These physicians are assisted in their work by legions of basic scientists, pharmacists, chemists, mechanical engineers, et.al. Many of these people are employed by the nation's medical schools. Much research is also funded by large pharmaceutical corporations who are strongly incentivized by the somewhat infinite largesse of profit obtainable from the invention of the right drug or the right device, profits well protected by the nation's patent laws and the federal legislature whom they donates scads of dollars to when they seek election and re-election, and re-election. In fact it is probably impossible to survive politically on the national stage without some good friends in big pharma. These huge drug companies as well as biotechs and medical device makers also employ cadres of scientists as well as teams of lawyers, accountants, administrative personnel and some generally wealthy people to sit on the boards of directors, people who know how to count money, protect money, and make more money in that they have done it before and that is what they do. Many of the bioscientists on the faculties of every one of our medical teaching institutions also hold positions in research, product development, never mind the boards of directors.

Thus it is capitalism that has fueled these revolutionary medical advances. I say this as a fact of reality despite my own politics which suggests that we as a people should create and contribute because there is need, because it is the right thing to do. I think a lot about this when I see a seven page hospital bill, look at the receipt from a corner pharmacy, have my eyes drop out when I see the new medical insurance premium rates, or see a patient declined for service because of the lack of insurance at all or even with insurance that they have paid a king's ransom for. You know, some minor service like chemotherapy for their cancer.

Capitalism is a lion with a huge difficult to satiate appetite.

There is also a ground war in this crusade. That is where the family physician's role comes into play. The fact that it is cardiovascular disease which makes us ill more than any other entity, cardiovascular disease which tends to kill us, cardiovascular disease which fills our nursing homes, cardiovascular disease which busts our wallets, the family doctor is strongly encouraged to make this a focus.

The cornerstone of our methodology has for generations been called the annual physical or more recently the health maintenance exam. This includes a thorough top to bottom exam, the bottom part of which can be interpreted literally. Patients will often arrive for this exam with a list of 27 problems or questions, the full discussion of each which might require review of a complete textbook.

The fundamental question of this going over might be voiced, "Well, Doc, how long am I going to live?" An appropriate question in that it is in fact a substantial part of what we do is to get a detailed grasp on the risk factors for cardiovascular disease. These are obvious to us in the sense that they constitute the worldview of modern medicine. They include the presence or absence of hypertension, the presence or absence of diabetes mellitus, the family history in detail, lipid levels - good cholesterol, bad cholesterol, total cholesterol, triglycerides. Looking at the individual's weight, diet, sodium intake, exercise habits or the lack thereof. Each of these issues requires a vast armamentarium of factual information and a poker player's hand of verbal skills and approaches to get inside the patient's head. This is not one size fits all. This is about knowing an individual in a deeply personal way, engendering a level of trust, and somehow promulgating a milieu of feasible ways to embark on meaningful change.

If the first three rules of a good golf swing are keep your head down, keep your head down, and keep your head down, there can be no doubt that the first three rules of general medical practice are don't smoke, don't smoke, don't smoke. I do not doubt that the discussion of cigarette smoking cessation is the single most time consuming item in the life of a family physician. It is nicotine not death that is our mortal enemy to be battled with at every juncture. It is nicotine that deprives so many of us of decent health, a chance at the enjoyment of life. Helping people to quit is a continuous war, a war which is relentless and must be approached dynamically with protean powers of persuasion.

Too much of what I know about the fierceness and deeply seated nature of nicotine I know from personal experience. My own total ingestion was one puff of a cigarette at age 19 though for a number of years I would enjoy a cigar at a ballgame or on the golf course or playing music. I still like the smell of a pipe or a cigar. There were other herbal inhalables that I was less averse to.

On the other hand, among the long and profound personal relationships in my life was Dad Long, a relationship that at first just came in the bargain with marrying Cindy but over the next several decades became its own source of enjoyment to me as we shared the love of his oldest daughter, the four daughters Cindy and I would have (four of his seven granddaughters after having three daughters and a son which probably went a ways to explain his special affection for his grandson Sam, though Sam was born pretty lovable in general. Dad Long and I also shared a passion for chasing a little white ball with names like Titleist and Pro-flight which we pursued with rugged determination and shared concentration of effort though poor Mr. Long did not have the full appreciation of hitting the ball anywhere near as many times per round as I did or with such interesting curves and caroms. I loved the man and we had a great time together.

Dad Long graduated high school early in the Second World War, precociously, not surprising given his astute natural intellect and then claimed an unofficial waver on his age to join the Navy and some overseas travel in the waters of the Pacific. He was never much on talking in detail

about his experiences but he did return to a life of marriage and family and home building with a serious habit of several packs of cigarettes per day, mostly unfiltered which caused significant pulmonary insufficiency at a young age and significant emphysema by the time he should have been enjoying many golden years on the golf course.

I had begun foisting the issue of why not to smoke on him early on when I was still a medical student with the vigor of the righteous, on my own and with Cindy's encouragement. He always listened attentively and respectfully. It was late in the game when years later Cindy and I were summonsed to Philadelphia where after a number of weeks of worsening shortness of breath and a refractory cough he had gone into respiratory failure and had been admitted to a hospital on an emergency basis. After a screaming streak to Phillie we arrived in time to find Dad on the cusp. Having done a large amount of pulmonology I was able to push for the right interventions and with due haste necessary to bring him from the brink. I stayed at his bedside straight through for the next several days as he convalesced. This included watching up close and personal what nicotine withdrawal actually looks like. The nausea, the tremor, the fear, the panic, the sweating, the sense of imminent disaster. Dad survived this and I never forgot a moment of it.

Most of the next ten years that he was able to live after that were with an oxygen tank in tow, many, many doctor visits and a lot of gasping, hawking, coughing, and general misery. I will never forget the moment toward his end when he looked me in the face and said tearfully, "I never thought I was going to pay for the smoking, but now I am, Big Time." Part of his legacy has been that I believe that the recitation of this story to many of my patients over the years has been of aide in helping many kindred spirits to successfully give it up. A week before his passing Dad Long was able to come to Massachusetts and have a dance in the hotel room which he wasn't physically able to leave with my daughter Marie, beautiful bride shortly to be who loved her grandfather greatly. I have always considered him to be a great man.

I met Myrtle Kosegarten in the Coronary Care Unit of Hillcrest Hospital. She was in the hyper-acute phase of an acute myocardial inferior wall infarction; in the current time she would have been transferred to a regional center for emergency catheterization and likely stent implantation. However, it was 1974 and we monitored, waited for the enzymes to come back to normal, and estimated the amount of myocardial damage.

Myrtle was a fifty-six year old woman hanging on to a fair amount of feminine prettiness who clearly was conscious of and attended to maintaining a fashionable appearance. She was stylish definitely, but her more prominent quality was a friendly outgoingness; she pretty well loved everyone and everyone loved her. Especially Herman, a GE engineer just a few years her senior. They rather adored each other. They were usually seen in each other's company, always with a lot of winks and giggling going on. It was unfortunate at that time that she had been smoking a pack of cigarettes a day since late adolescence, typical and suave for her generation.

I had a serious talk with her about the relationship between cigarette smoking and coronary artery disease. She never smoked another cigarette.

Today she remains a patient of mine at 95 still fully ambulatory, cognitively intact as we say, good eyes, fair ears (you have to speak up to her a little) and a sense of optimistic joyfulness that has never waned - she still laughs happily enough at even slightly funny comments.

My anticipation of her grief at the loss of her Herman two years ago also a patient of mine for forty plus years always motivated me to keep him going even as he gradually declined through his nineties, his lifelong tendency to anxiety magnifying with the aging of his brain. When he did pass at 98, though I am sure Myrtle still misses him, she has not wavered from her joyful ways.

She still does not smoke and has no evidence whatsoever of cardiac disease.

Last Christmas she had delivered to me the Westinghouse electric toaster which she and Herman had received as a wedding present in 1942 and which had worked well for them through many years of tea and toast. It remains in perfect shiny condition, mint. She wanted me to have it. I can only hope that the care I have given her is in the same league with the care she and Herman gave that toaster which now sits proudly in its place on our kitchen counter. For me it will always be a living metaphor for the value of taking good care of things, the beauty of long marriages, and the value of not smoking.

Frank Szelest is the salt of the earth.

I first met him in circumstances similar to Myrtle Kosegarten, admitted to the Coronary Care Unit also in 1974 on an emergency basis in the throes of acute myocardial infarction. He stabilized rapidly and was soon ready for discharge without complications, just lacking the horsepower of a chunk of his myocardium. He was also a heavy smoker and had telescoped into his 42 year old vital male body fifty pack years of cigarettes.

I pointed out to him the prognostic implications of continued smoking and he responded with something like, "Okay, Doc thanks for telling me that." He never smoked another cigarette and I have had the privilege and enjoyment of taking care of him for the ensuing four decades.

I always loved the fact that for forty years Frank got up at three in the morning to get to the dairy for loading up to deliver milk before the kids left for school all over Pittsfield, door to door, never missing a day. For all of these years his hairstyle, his sauntering walk, his easy smile, and his workingman wardrobe have been invariant.

Now in his mid-70's he is vitally healthy, continuous with easy words of kindness and spends most of his time toting his grandchildren about town to ballgames and practices. And once a year he and his wife take a cruise to the Caribbean.

His children have all grown to responsible citizenship. None of his grandchildren have ever smoked he proudly told me. If you would like to meet him you can go the Highland Restaurant on Tuesdays where he will be eating spaghetti at about six p.m.

The basic fund of medical information which we use in this war on cardiovascular disease is something which I find interesting, definitely useful and necessary, but it is the area of coming to grips with the vagaries and life challenges of every individual who comes before you is where I find medicine intriguing and potentially greatly satisfying, often if not always.

You come to a point in each exam where it comes down to, "Well, Doc, how am I doing?"

This lead to questions like well how do you think you're doing, what do you really want out of your life, how long do you want to live, why and wherefore, what happens when you do come to an end, and what do you what that to look like. More interestingly what happens after this particular journey ceases. What is of the greatest importance in the meantime?

One such conversation comes to mind. Eleanor now climbing into her upper eighties had been a friend and co-parishioner long before she had ever become a patient. She will always appear in my mind as the statuesque lady always with a French twist and a chiffon scarf in the front row of the choir alto section at The First Church and twice a year addressing the congregation on one of her favorite "charities", the blueberry festival in the Spring and the Harvest Festival in the Fall. Her husband Tom was a professional church organist of some renown. His religion I think was first and foremost the organ and specific church affiliation more of a secondary matter. They both carried an aura of old time Yankee with an air of quality education, deep respect for manners and proper syntax, sophisticated humor. They never had children.

When she became a patient things had become more complicated with the exigencies of mutually failing memory function and the lack of a next generation to look after their needs. This accelerated over the next few years during which her office visits became more frequent before rather abruptly disappearing altogether, during which time the church activities became a matter of past tense. I never once heard about any calls or visits from co-worshipers. Tom ended up placed in an extended care facility which depleted their limited resources in quick order.

It was late in this context when Eleanor and I got into it, that is trying to come up with some thoughts and rationalizations that might make her stressful circumstances a bit easier to struggle along with. For some reason I presented her with the speculative question of what does she suppose happens when it is all over and done with? Given her long and dedicated service to our former place of worship I was a bit surprised when she responded succinctly with a single term - "HUBRIS." I think a sort of choked, and muttered something like, "Pardon me?" She again responded in kind - Hubris - which made me wonder aloud, "And what was all that church going about?" To which responded simply and without a hint of malice or regret, "Well, I just thought that was a fine bunch of people to be associated with. I personally at least feel very much that way about Eleanor.

All of these subjects and questions are fair game and it is the conversations I have around these issues which make medicine a source of immeasurable fascination, a ceaseless intellectual and spiritual journey, and a fountain of infinite personal reward, probably only surpassed by trying to be a good husband, a good father, very much at the core of the meaning of my own life. I get to be a philosopher, a spiritual guide, a shaman, a confessor, a granter of peace and wisdom. What a great job.

Thus it is to my patients that I owe my deepest gratitudes.

THE BIRDCOUNTER

Monomoy rises at the horizon of a summer morning,
the sands lose their moisture to the first touch of sun,
beach grass awakens from the blackness of night-
emerging green, fragrant.
The song is one of silence,
broken only by the splash of the ocean,
against the island's delicate rim,
and the rising symphony
of the morning calls
of a million birds
and the soft steps upon the sand
of one man
come to count each one:
The Birdcounter.
Slowly, deliberately, and alone,
he traverses the island step after step,
wizened hands grasping tripod and lens,
squinting aged eyes ready to focus once more
at his counting station
at the edge of the wetlands,
which he could easily call his own,
the nursery and playground of the million birds,
which he could easily also call his own,
ready to count into and through the torpid heat of the day,
ready to count,
not for himself,
but rather for each of us,
for everyman,
for every one of us,

who walks and prays on this earth,
beholden to its bounty,
beholden to its creator.

Now far from that island
at the edge of winter,
the New England mountains I love,
once again stripped bare,
braced to endure the cold,
I also am drawn to count.
The complexities of this human life.
The reality of physical pain, suffering.
The frailty of human conviction.
The measured limits of faith.
I count out the last breaths of a dying man.
I count to the last beat of the heart,
my hand on his chest, my eyes peering into his own.
I understand that each of his days
were long ago counted and numbered,
as are also my own.
And I pray for the courage that also understands,
that for each act of treachery,
there can be a greater act of redemption;
that for each stabbing time of loss,
there can be a far greater time of awakening;
that for each death,
there will certainly one day be another born.
Heading home,
needing to rest before dawn,
I remember the Birdcounter,
and I whisper to him across the sky,
please don't forget to count,
for all of us,
until one day we are free,
to count for ourselves.

9

ADDICTIVE ILLNESS

Higher and Higher
JACKIE WILSON

ON THE SAME Scotland circumlocution which Cindy and I made in 2012, on one sunny summer's midday we found ourselves at the foot of ye olde Ben Nevus, the old sod's most majestic peak. We parked our rental car in an area designed to serve as a base for aspiring Ben Nevus conquerors. The majestic mountain with its step like chain of antecedents stood before us with its well-trodden trekway beckoning like the Yellow Brick Road to the Emerald City of Oz, mysterious and rich with beauty in the distant mist. I often have dreamed of the mist, the explanation for which I usually perceived as a pathway to a higher enlightenment, perhaps even having a bearing on our eventual post-corporeal journey. On this occasion we had in mind the intention of a serious hike, seeing some great views, snapping a few sheep and goat photos, accomplishing some aerobic exercise. Attaining the peak was not our goal.

This recollection comes to mind as a good enough metaphor for my own attitude on the subject of substances and drugs - it's safer being an interested observer at the base camp than being an apex seeker. The recollection also serves as a metaphor for the prospect on embarking on composing a consolidation of my thoughts and experiences on the general subject of addictive illness. It's a definite mountain climb.

The practice of family medicine in the current era is embroiled in the complex matrix and vicious tentacles of these illnesses just as the whole of our society, the whole of our families is mired like a cowboy in quicksand. It behooves any physician intent on having an impact in their community as a positive force against human pain and suffering to master a level of sophistication and expertise in this area.

I have already vented at length on the central role of cigarette smoking in the pathogenesis of cardiovascular disease, pulmonary disease, neoplastic disease in general. Suffice it to say that with our staff and colleagues and in our documentation we use the terms cigarette smoking and nicotine addiction rather interchangeably, i.e. as one disease. We probably spend, quite appropriately, as much time on identifying nicotine addiction, educating on this subject and doing smoking cessation counseling as any other issue in our daily mission. This time well spent can clearly promote in the long run better health for every given individual with genuine benefit as well for their families and communities.

This exam room conversation around smoking certainly can become redundant and tiresome. I sometimes perceive an annoying echo in my head when I launch into this, but it is a war and there can be no letup. An especially common projection at least is that patients in general must be astonished at the preoccupation medical professionals appear to have on the matter. Nevertheless it is truly almost impossible to exaggerate the significance of smoking - the total amount of disease which is directly connected to smoking is beyond statistical measure, which makes the human toll in lost life and liberty even more beyond our ken. I can think easily and readily of enumerable individuals, men and women, whom I have cared for over decades who have lived the life of the widow - years of loneliness, eating solitary meals, sleeping alone, living off of the continuously fading memory of the love of their lives - their life partners having passed away at young ages of malignancies directly related to the smoking habit.

Barbara Seddon is a woman who has been well known to me over many years, nearly my same age now as she was when we first met forty years ago, at that time to attend to her fairly severe asthma. She has always been an intellectually bright individual, prettier than most, and wittier than your average Joe. She grew up in a jazz household, her father broadcasting jazz program years ago out of Albany and indoctrinating his daughter on the subject. She continues to promote modern jazz locally. She once gave me a present of some private stock CD's of her dad conversing philosophically with Duke Ellington; remarkable, a little like listening to the voice of God.

I also for many years took care of her husband Charlie, also very much an affable sort with legions of loyal customers for his contracting business; people liked Charlie and liked his work equally. They were high school sweethearts and had four kids together, most with fiery red hair. Charlie was blessed with the handsome good looks of a high school quarterback and a sincere happy enough smile, but was nobody's fool. He knew what a day's work looked like and was not afraid of doing many, many. Usually while he was at work he had a cigarette hanging from his lips or on the edge of the workbench.

This all worked beautifully for this All American family until ten years ago when an x-ray done because of a nagging cough showed an irregularly marginated mass in his right upper lobe. Two-years later he died after failing treatment with some gruesome chemotherapy. Barbara's golden years prospects changed from patiently waiting for the 40th and the 50th and the 60th wedding anniversaries with the love of her life to just missing him, every second of every day as the years drag on. She tries. She has struggled valiantly but when this happens part of what you are is gone. When I speak with Barbara I feel Charlie's absence in every word out of her mouth.

My patient Ellie cleans houses. And works at the local Big Y in the delicatessen where she bakes bread and pastries for half of the town. Neither is easy work but she does both joyfully with a friendly smile and the willingness to laugh at any good joke that she is told. She continues with both jobs now at 75, slightly frail and osteopenic, but also trim and petite, but usually quite exhausted. Her "ladies" as she calls them and her Big Y customers will not allow her to retire. Her heartbeat is now irregular at times.

Her life was not always that of a spinster. There once was a guy named Tony. With whom Ellie fell permanently in love with as a teenager. She was cute and a little shy but Tony was more the bad boy who loved to lean against his '57 Chevy at the drive-in on summer nights, his luscious black locks combed straight back (about every eight minutes), his tee shirt sleeves rolled up to emphasize some biceps. I met him when I was 25 to his 35 and we got along fine. Except for the fact that he developed lung cancer before he was forty and died in six months. For the 35 years which I have known Ellie, if you say the word "Tony" a twinkle will come to her eye and she will say something like, "Yeah, he was a hot ticket." There has never been another.

Ruth Gentry is now in her mid-80's, as stern of a woman as you might want to know. She supports herself on Social Security and by doing people's taxes. I am sure with great precision and a firm grasp on current codes and regulations. I know of no other four foot eleven, eighty-eight pound tiger that I would less like to scramble with. I have taken care of her since 1974 though the vast majority of our time together has been Ruth establishing repeatedly who is the boss. Which I have no argument with. And telling me what is actually wrong with her and what she should do about it. This method saves work actually. Her life was not always without humor or companionship. Her husband Jimmy also became a patient of mine when she sent him over to get checked out. He was funny, personable, good looking, even if a bit afraid of his wife. He liked everyone and everyone liked him until five years later in his early forties when he succumbed to a sudden heart attack, an unpredictable occurrence except for his previous chain-smoking. Ruth took this event to be nothing more than the calculable outcome of his smoking but on a deeper level I believe that she has been a bit mad at the world ever since. At least I have never seen her in a good mood. We sort of love and admire each other from the safety of distance. Ruth has always made it easier for me to understand why the owners of pit bulls find them adorable.

Bonnie Lennon Leach is something of a legend locally. She is now in her fifties, but as a high school student she did buzz her brother Robert's motorcycle in one end of Wahconah High School and out the other full throttle and then wait outside for the police to arrive. Robert was also a patient of mine. He had returned from combat service in Viet Nam unfortunately with one arm blown off. He was in fact one hell of a nice guy, became a leader of the local Viet Nam Vets, and led many parades. I had been a conscientious objector but we definitely liked each other and got along fine. Our conversations always included how he was a heavy cigarette smoker and that was a serious threat to his health. At 38 he developed lung cancer and died about as quickly as his arm had been shot off.

Bonnie as well as her adorably sweet husband Steve and their many kids and grandkids remain patients of ours to this day. Salt of the earth. "We have a lot of tomatoes. Do you want some? And here's some squash." They are great. But there have been many times when it would have been helpful for Bonnie for Robert to have been there. She still misses him thirty years later, as do many others in Pittsfield, myself included.

Thank you cigarettes.

I could tell a hundred of these stories. Alone in an exam room with a cigarette smoking patient it is usually only necessary to refer to the patient in the next room to have a frame of reference for the ravages of smoking. How can a sane person not hate this addiction?

Let me begin the discussion of what we do about his by explaining in fact my own intensity on the subject. A successful attempt to promote cessation begins with absolving the patient from any sense of being judged - morally or personally. I language to the person that it is the damage done by the habit that we disdain, not the person smoking. Hate the sin, love the sinner. I remind myself from the outset that the patient I am dealing with is already well aware of the foolishness and danger of the habit. That they are already probably feeling guilty enough. Their children and grandchildren and husband or wife (if they don't smoke themselves) have probably already been harassing them. In this day and age most smokers would prefer to not smoke. It is just a matter of getting from Point A to Point B. I love the awakened sense of personal pride and satisfaction that successful quitters are imbued with.

In fact I often point out to them that anyone who has successfully detoxed from nicotine once and for all can overcome anything that they are likely to be challenged with, that they can climb any mountain (even Ben Nevus) by using the same commitment and method.

The casual illness - bronchitis, a sinus infection, pneumonia - usually easily and quickly treatable can provide a starting point to begin the discussion. The health maintenance physical also obviously provides a fair game format. I often will point out to folks that smoking is the only black mark on their health record, the only issue standing between them and an open field. I emphasize that many millions of people have been able to quit. And that most of those people at one time didn't think they could.

Mostly people are very open and appreciative of this conversation, even hard core smokers. They can sense a doctor's genuine concern and react to the lack of judgment. If someone really doesn't want to hear it, save your ammunition for a better time. Though I will say those particular addicts usually end up paying big time sooner or later.

I then make a case as persuasively as I can that the first step is once and for all deciding that it can be done. I try to get the patient to visualize themselves as a nonsmoker, always a welcome image. I emphasize that (1) believing that you can do it and (2) that you are going to do it are all that matters. The rest is detail. If a caring physician can get the smoker to that point by meaning it and by finding the appropriate unique words which a given individual can hear, there is no reason not to succeed steadily and join with the patient in the joy of their success. And also save a lot of lives. The fact that no two dialogs are the same is a big part of the satisfaction, far from redundant or boring. If there is art in medicine it is in finding these words.

The uniqueness of this shared process, the fact that you are building a bridge for a good person to reach the land of good health is a lot like a successfully executed piece of jazz improvisation. Not that it is about the doctor's ego but knowing that a patient you really like has successfully made a life changing leap largely because they knew you were just not going away can be incredibly rewarding. This leap which I have had the good fortune to experience too many times to count tends to self-motivate, in fact to induce the desire to never stop getting better at it.

The process of helping a patient overcome any addiction is some strange combination of the mysterious magic of the white coat (which I have never worn) in some carefully measured connection with the patient, person to person, devoid of medical authoritarianism. The fact that I can't completely understand or explain the nature of this transaction always makes it for me a little bit of magic.

Once again to reiterate I have always seen the details of how to quit smoking to be somewhat moot - nicotine replacement products, puffers, gum, patches, whatever I have never pushed in that the logic of replacing a drug with the same drug is a stretch, especially nowadays when more smokers are quitting from a lower dose starting place. Wellbutrin (Buproprion) may well be the pick of the litter when you are facing a stormy withdrawal reaction. Chantix can do it but has tricky side effects. The bottom line remains that partnership with the patient and that difficult to explain lending library dance of lending same faith and hope to another person until they don't need it anymore lies at the heart of the matter.

And that's it for addictive issues.

I wish.

The phenomenon of the addictive personality.

You do come across individuals who can and will become addicted to anything and over time I have seen one of everything. I visualize that there exists in each of us a spectrum very much DNA determined and I mean by a precise number of toxic sites, and that where you fall on that spectrum will predict your likelihood of dealing with an addiction along the way. I also superimpose on that idea the entire aura of social, parenting, economic qualities and experiences with potential to draw out and actualize addictiveness. If you have all of the addiction DNA sites on your own little chromosomal strands hang on for a wild ride. If your life experience and circumstances are also dysfunctional, then head for an ashram or some South Sea island where fruit cannot be fermented.

I recently lost a patient, Mr. Robert Daley, at age 57 to alcoholism after a battle which I shared in as his Secretary of State over his entire adulthood which included approximately two hundred detox admissions, a dozen or so incarcerations, a couple dozen psych admissions, and an occasional suicide gesture. The strange thing was that when not drinking he could readily be engaged in sincere intellectually sophisticated dialog on the nature of addiction and strategizing to attain sobriety which over the years he got better and better at. Several times we were able to look forward to celebrating one year anniversaries and his life in general would go well for those periods.

Robert was boyishly handsome, charming, and absolutely no judge of danger which would often get him into situations where he would get the shit kicked out of him by some more violent alcoholics. His death came as no surprise as he had long defied the odds. This did not prevent the shedding of a few heartfelt tears reflecting on his life with his surviving sister Linda, also a patient, also an alcoholic, as is virtually every member of this struggling family for several generations. Linda said to me when we last spoke, "Bobby liked you a lot." I indicated that to be mutual and that I missed him.

Daniel A. has the kind of good looks in the U.S Male that you look for on the cover of G.Q. or whatever or maybe an NFL draft pick for quarterback. And he is highly intelligent, appropriate in social context, well-mannered, qualities which he shares with all of his family members. His father runs a successful local real estate business. Michael has also achieved a streak of the highest blood alcohol levels I have ever seen. Damndest thing. You can have an intelligent, productive conversation with him at four in the afternoon, freshly barbered and in a freshly ironed business shirt and at seven- thirty get a call about him from the emergency unit with a blood alcohol level through the ceiling - over and over and over again. His parents who love him and would give their own lives for his survival have had the impossible task of accepting that a fatal overdose was not beyond the range of the possible. Fortunately the acuteness of that fear has dimmed as Daniel has done major recovery work.

Talk about the need for a higher power. Not only does Daniel have in common with other alcoholics the lack of a shutoff switch, he seems to have some kind of turbo-charged crank it up switch stuck in his brain - some kind of demand which only alcohol can sate. Wild.

His sister Michele is also a patient and also an All American with a broad smile and sophisticated manner. In early adulthood she took off for the West Coast and became enmeshed in an inner city drug culture - cocaine, speed, heroine, you name it, usually in combinations. This led her to the acquaintanceship of some bad people and major squalor from which she was only extricated by the grace of God. She is now at the top of her nursing school class and celebrating three years of grateful recovery in AA and goes to a whole lot of meetings. Her future seems to lack any limits.

So what is it all about?

Basically we are a species which universally harbors a potential for addiction to mind altering substances that is as old as time. I do not believe that these people have a character weakness or defect in that in sobriety they are if anything better than most of us - kind, sensitive, generous. I think the phenomenon is for the most part hardwired which makes it perhaps less mysterious and less given to esoteric philosophic rambling explanations but just basically a part of what we are. Each generation seems to have the need to concoct its own culture of drugs of choice but as Janis Joplin said famously on "Pearl," "Shit, man, it's all the same God damned thing." She was pretty stoned at the time, but I do think she was referring to the nineteen different drugs in her system. Man she could sing.

My personal experience.

Alcohol has been a part of my life's experience.

Actually since the day I was born in that my mother's worldview and personality though a total teetotaler was formed largely by the cauldron of my grandfather's alcoholism. During my own coming of age and even college years' alcohol wasn't much in sight but this was largely due to my generational bias toward marijuana which was extant. I did enjoy and using the word fuck a lot, eating brownies, listening to Pink Floyd, etc. That was all over at least for me when Ronald Reagan became President and I declared an official end to my childhood.

After then we developed a sort of social life that included an unending sequence of dinner parties usually loosened a little with white wine ("Oh, doesn't that have a wonderful bouquet," and all that bullshit.) This was fairly family friendly and we also at one point took dance lessons and looked high and low for places to practice our steps. My own virtuosity on the dance floor was usually enhanced by two (or four) Tom Collins or whatever. We had fun. I never heard from a friend any comment on my own dosage and they were the leaders of the legal, medical, clerical communities so they must know something. I was always a little conscious about being careful with alcohol but never had a serious concern.

Then the strangest thing happened.

My own shutoff valve went kaput.

Briefly at a restaurant dinner attended by a dozen or so good friends, a bit much wine was ordered, the wasting of which violated my own Scottish sense of frugality. The next day I was concerned. What was that about?

That was in the autumn; I didn't drink for a few months.

Then there was a New Year's Eve party at a big house on a hill sort of a frat party for the Over the Hill Gang. The need to master a few double flips and cartwheels on the dance floor eventuated in too many paper cups of wine. Unfortunately the night ended badly (very badly) with my wife kindly and generously offering the opinion that I did not seem to be safe with alcohol, a conclusion which I had already arrived at. That was my last drink, soon to be twenty years ago and my only feelings toward the aroma, appearance, and socialization around Etoh have been an ongoing repugnance.

That's my story and I'm sticking to it though additions or elaborations are fair game. For myself my own blame and shame has always been quite enough, thank you. When I did do my own fourth step after doing a thorough and honest self-examination, I did find that most of the harm my own drinking had done was to me. Looking in life at what pain you may have caused a spouse or children I have to say is about as tough a chore as any. Whatever I could have done differently I have tried to make up for.

But that does bring up the subject of the single most miraculous medical breakthrough of the Twentieth Century to segue from my troubles such as they were. After the above Olde Land Syne debacle I did decide to seek counsel and advice at a Massachusetts Medical Society organization designed for the purpose. In fact Cindy made their phone number available to me. This required a little travel but did enable me to get a good start on the road to recovery and meet some rather remarkable individuals, many of whom I still think back on occasionally who told some remarkable stories. Which I will not share. But don't ever say that doctors are boring.

The fundamental entrenchment of the twelve step process in this group was not surprising to me as I had studied it in an academic way and had found it useful in working with alcoholics and drug addicts for years but what had been academic became more literal.

After my first meeting which I have to say was a bit surrealistic I did have an interchange with a very wise and substantially recovered prime mover of the group and his parting words to me were that if I were to drink over the weekend to call him and he would set up some inpatient care. To express how little of a craving I had for any form of alcohol at that point would be difficult but it did occur to me that it would always be presumed by program people in general that I was doing some minimizing. For the record there were two times in my life when I felt out of control with alcohol alluded to above, only rarely drank excessively, never drank habitually, and for the twenty years since have found the amount of drinking in my immediate social milieu to be very much in the range of what I knew I could not deal with. I have always seen that abhorrence as a higher power gift and have often wished it was easier to share. It is rarely difficult to make the case that most situational enjoyments, the quality of most relationships, or much else of anything is improved by a drug effect. I pledged at that time to dedicate myself to being spiritually honest and sober and to be of as much help to others as I possibly could. The sight and aroma of alcohol reinforces that for me. Not that I find the occasional waft of marijuana in the air at a concert or whatever totally unpalatable as long as it is someone else's brain doing the drifting away.

Thus the miracle of the Twelve Steps.

1. We admitted that we were powerless.
2. Believe in a power greater than ourselves.
3. Turn our will over to that higher power.
4. Made a searching inventory of ourselves.

5. Admitted our wrongs.

6. Prepared ourselves to have them removed.

7. Asked our higher power to remove our shortcomings.

8. Made a list of whom we have injured

9. Made amends.

10. Admit it when you screw up.

11. Get closer to the sacred.

12. Give back whatever you can.

Paraphrased.

Simple as that.

You can add to that model the genius of the Serenity Prayer as defined by:

God grant me the serenity to accept the things I cannot change,
the courage to change the things I can,
and the wisdom to know the difference.

Helps a lot.

And for me, please add the New Testament scriptural admonition of Jesus Christ when asked "and how then Master shall we pray?" "Pray without ceasing."

Which I have always taken to mean that the best aspiration which we can set our human sights on is to allow every breath, every thought, every word take on the sanctity of prayer. Striving for that ideal has been returned to me infinitely in the largesse of what I might call miracle awareness - in music, in the whole of nature, in the faces, kindnesses, heroisms of the human race surrounding me. That and the very useful medical definition of alcoholism. "When the patient drinks more than the doctor." have always served me well in having some radar for the disease. It is in almost every family somewhere - the desire and capacity to be of service to suffering individuals is more of a gift than a responsibility.

Trust me, it is everywhere.

Then of course there is heroin, narcotic pills - readily available at your local emergency room or pain clinic. Good Old Marijuana, designer drugs, and to mention the gamut of sex and love addictions and perhaps the most lethal of all - gambling addiction - quite generally lethal or at least likely to create the need for a change of address, perhaps to somewhere in Argentina.

A short qualifier on the subject of substance abuse medical care.

Even making a leap into the land of recovery, I was never enamored with the idea that it was the doctor's responsibility to disaffect every individual who likes to drink or drug from the notion. In fact it has been my personal experience that the vast majority of that population will continue along their chosen paths until some likely premature early demise. In my own extended group of friends whom Cindy and I cherish I know of no other single individual who does not drink "at all" and likewise no individual who is "in recovery." Not that it is my business and in fact part of living sober is developing obliviousness to the behaviors around you unless someone seeks feedback or help. But most drinkers keep on drinking. I have rarely attended a twelve step meeting without the passing thought that while this handful of people are sitting praying together and sharing there are a whole lot more out in the great out there doing their thing. What is the ratio? Blank to one. I like to analyze things mathematically and this math tells me that recovery is a gift granted to a fortunate few, which has always made it easier for me to get my mind around the idea of an involved divinely endowed higher power. I never chose to make the twelve steps into a religion. It has always worked better for me as one way among many to solve problems and look at life but there is indeed a wealth of miracle woven through those steps and what they can do in an individual's life. I have been fortunate to witness this in the paths of a large number of recovering souls and the lives they touch.

To broaden the discussion further, I already floated a few theories about sexual proclivities, standard and aberrant, but this does have a niche in addictive illness.

My long anthropologic view of sexuality is that nature and/or God endowed us with these drives as for purposes of procreation and thus survival, one part of the very grand scheme which we call the balance of nature. The ubiquitous nature of reproductive functions across the phyla of both plant and animal does not tend to argue absolutely for either prime source.

I suspect that what we call normal though this concept alone has never ceased to evolve through the ages, especially so in the modern era of rapid-fire social change, is at its core designed to serve a survival function. And what we choose to look at as aberrancies are just false starts or alterations on the template - perhaps a growth and development twist or turn or just a DNA sequence gone awry.

I am certain that the difficulty which we have had historically with understanding homosexuality is rather purely defined by chromosomal dictate will be looked at by future generations as quaint, akin to why Christopher Columbus was worried about his boats dropping off the edge of the planet, well actually the world at that time. As I think about it three tall ships with all male crews setting sail across the Atlantic for Miami Beach was probably not the worst job for a bunch of gay guys at the time. Neither do I doubt that in a few hundred years the progeny of Senator Michelle Bachman will still be determined to proscribe same gender libido as the wrath of God.

But fetishes, like being aroused by envisioning women's leather gloves or the sensation of the whack of a belt on your hindquarters might be more likely related to an early childhood experience with a sadistic mother or father or aunt or uncle or cartoon character. Who knows? Though I expect that having affairs serially, obsession with nasty sex - pornography, prostitution, whatever - might have more to do with a hypothalamic or limbic lobe shutoff circuit breaker or something of the sort. We will eventually know.

If some of us don't know that three dozen doughnuts might not be enough even if the scale said four hundred that morning or that one more snort, or pop, or injection, or nightcap when you already forgot who the first President was a few hours before, then why not a similar mechanism for knowing how much sex is enough or what sexual behavior is pragmatic and appropriate for the successful preservation of your intimate relationship as well as your species.

One of the sadnesses of these aberrancies is that even for those who might choose some help, there is little available. Psychiatry? Sorry, waste of time. Some would argue. Drugs? Probably more likely to make things worse. And try adding a twelve step program for sexual addiction to your resume before you apply for your next job.

Likewise the only modality which I have ever seen having a lasting impact on food addiction is Overeaters Anonymous, also lacking in availability in most areas and sadly only much good to overeaters with the spiritual and intellectual tools necessary to bene-fit. I have attended a few OA meetings and was only slightly surprised that the waistlines there were probably better than at the gym. No surprise that the economically deprived who live with morbid obesity usually die from morbid obesity at a young age. It's no good to be poor but at least if you are fat and poor neither will last as long.

Twelve step programs for gamblers? Don't bother looking. They have already had their kneecaps shot off and that didn't help. Actually the members at AA and NA meetings who are lacking kneecaps are really there for gambling addiction.

So let's see. Let's add this all up.

That leaves two eunuch monks in a cave in Tibet, three mechanical engineers in Birmingham, Alabama, with checkered bow ties and pressed short sleeve white shirts from Sears with vinyl pocket savers, four goatherds wandering the deserts of eastern Iran, and five partridges in a pear tree and we have the total number of non-addicted human beings on the planet. Plus one church lady in Minnesota knitting mittens for the poor. And don't be surprised if you find out that the goatherds are doing some toking while the Mullah isn't watching. And the goats probably should watch each other backs to be on the safe side as well.

Thus my basic conclusion that addiction is in the longest view a fundamental part of the human condition. How we deal with it unfortunately has rather infinite consequences for lost years of life for the afflicted individual, wars between nations fought over the commerce of alcohol and drugs, street crime, gang warfare, crime in general - robbing convenience stores and killing girlfriends - automobile and motorcycle deaths on the highway, and many manner of forms of brain damage, escalation of the divorce rate, abandonment of the love and care of children, to name a few.

Here's your quiz on addictive illness.

I have seen Beckett's Happy Days, Endgame, and Waiting for Godot a total of about fifteen times.

This drives my wife a little crazy.

Can you see why?

A. Why do I do it?

B. Why it drives he crazy?

Talk amongst yourselves.

Minor footnote.

There is not a single malady amongst all of the above that I have not at one time or another had the experience in my work as a physician of engaging with a patient on a soul level and with both honor and fascination and great reward witnessed astonishing human growth and change.

If addictive illness is in the final analysis emblematic of the human experience and a twelve step way of looking at the world - recognition of powerlessness, seeking a higher power, asking redemption, living in humility and gratitude, praying for grace - offers genuine hope - then a doctor can be the bridge to a better life.

Awesome.

I get to be this bridge, every single day.

10

SPECIAL CASES

Richard Gaudette

RICHARD GAUDETTE BECAME a patient of mine during my first week in practice. The emptying out of the "mental hospitals "which for eons had been the dumping grounds of society's rejects, the severely or even moderately retarded, and chronically psychotic, those afflicted with bizarre syndromes with names and without names, was in the process of rapidly hitting full swing. The new community-based tier of social service workers created to facilitate this process and support the outcome was in need of physicians open minded about taking care of the medical needs of these folks. Which in Pittsfield, Massachusetts, 1974 was me and for the next 40 years Family Practice Associates in all of its incarnations.

It was fortunate that I was still infiltrated with the newbie's discipline of beginning with the taking of a thorough past medical history. Richard's own life history carried about the same likelihood of success as mining for gold successfully in Northern California in 1849 or finding a newly discovered copy of the Dead Sea Scrolls already translated into modern English. His abdominal wall was in fact reminiscent of some type of Sanskrit code, the crisscrossing and crosshatching s on his abdomen told the tale of what was a repeated series of 26 surgical procedures stretching over his lifetime until he was able to fly the coop at age 32. He clearly had been the subject of some get some experience beach blanket bingo for some surgical training program.

From the time of his arrival in Pittsfield until his passing two decades later he never underwent another surgical procedure.

This medical profession abuse of his innocence showed no sign of resentment in the platonically friendly smile which embossed his not without cuteness demeanor always. He arrived with the countenance and mannerisms of your average 12-year-old All American boy and never seemed to age beyond that. This docile and benign demeanor was accentuated by the Mickey Mantle blondness of his always neatly cropped hair as well as the fact that he had undergone orchiectomy at some distant unspecified point in the past. His actual mental age was closer to seven or eight which made him an ideal playmate for our daughters Elizabeth and Amy who loved to play with Richard in the back yard as 5 or 10 minutes of leaf raking would be interspersed with a couple or three hours of trucks in the sandbox, picking dandelions, dressing up funny.

On one such occasion in the backyard Richard revealed to me the sacred secret as to why he never was seen without a comic book extruding from the back pocket of his hiked up beige khakis what I previously took as a statement as to his taste in the world of literature. He revealed to me this to be a much more practical calcula-tion. Richard did suffer from severe irritable bowel symptoms secondary to his many surgical procedures. On one such occasion upon heading to the John with a sense of emergency Richard smiled at me, reaching for his, comic book and saying in a private moment of sharing, "You know Docca Talo you nevah know when you may run out of toilet paper. "

In addition to the Taylor's, Richard was beloved in our community and a com-mon site on our city streets. At some point the retarded citizens' folks endowed him with a specially appointed three wheel bicycle with a large carrying baggage con-tainer with which Richard could thoroughly navigate all of the byways of our beloved village. Eventually his eternal smile and the diligence with which he ran up more miles on that contraption than the average 1964 Dodge won the citizens of Pittsfield over to a love of Richard.

I also recall Richard in the middle of a busy no catching up day in my office one mid-afternoon when he absolutely had to tell me the story of his morning's activities. I paused to listen to him. It seems he was in the local Berkshire bus going on his usual route, well known to the other regular passengers and the usual driver, when he took notice of smoke and flames emanating from a trashcan at the Park Square corner stop. He attempted to alert the other passengers and the bus driver to this conflagration outside the windows of the bus but was admonished to sit down and behave if he wanted to be allowed to ride on the bus, not once but twice. He was vindicated shortly thereafter when the fire truck came streaming around the corner. With a tear in his eye he finished with a single heartfelt statement, "You know Docca Talo, just cause a person is tawded does not mean they are stupid." It is with a similar tear in my own eye that I remember the goodness of this wonderful human being. I wrote a letter on Richard's passing to our local Berkshire Eagle editor and ended with a statement: "We all learned far more from Richard than he could ever learn from us." I stand by that statement now with years gone by and do not doubt that in some future incarnation Richard will be the first Fire him Chief of a low and I are her in a no after at work on Wednesday major American city with a PhD in philosophy.

Bill Strong

Bill Strong was also an early patient in the office. Exactly how he got my name I have no clue. At his first visit he just gave his address as Becket Mountain. He had no phone number. It emerged later that he was also known in the local environs as the Mountain Man or simply "the Woodchopper ". Others questioned his actual existence. There was a rumor of an estranged brother with whom I never had any contact. I think I prefer to consider it pure fate that he wandered in and chose me as his doctor. Maybe he was just due for his half century checkup. He was already in his 70s which was long before the ninth inning had become the seventh inning. Strong was a great name for him in that his lean body mass was strapped with well-toned sinews at every turn and his hands though blackened with coal tar and thickened by story of long years of hard work were at the same time both strong and gentle. He favored the clothing of heavy woolen work clothes. I never saw winter or summer without wearing a heavy Navy overshirt, drenched with the after burn of coal tar which I eventually learn he used for light, heat, and cooking. In addition to sturdy clothing he also had a fondness for Cindy who welcomed him to our office doing our reception duties. I think he had more total time with her than I ever did. I also think he was especially attracted to her interest and predilection for organic foods and gardening which the shared in common. He in fact grew all of his own food.

I also think he was somewhat attracted to her inside and outside beauties, not surprising in that it had been about five decades since he had had a conversation with a lady. In fact he eventually shared with me that it was the wake of a failed romantic relationship with another young lady upon returning from World War II many years previously that had sent him up on the Mountain supine, no pun intended.

I will not forget the blissful sun drenched October afternoon that Cindy and I and Amy and Elizabeth responded to Bill's invitation to visit him at his abode, an invitation that came only after we had become fast and close.

He had drawn a map.

Which we tried to follow assiduously, though most of the markings of trails were long abandoned hunting and utility trails and were much overgrown. I remember we did forge one stream in our Volkswagen van which I was not at all certain would be re- traceable. . We finally parked and trekked the last mile, literally following markings on certain trees which he had delineated on his map.

And then we entered the Magic Kingdom. Our way was helped by the fact that he had cleared an open meadow, cleared with his own strong hands, creating a rich tunnel of sunlight which guided us. He gave Cindy and I and our two young children with all eight of our eyes widened to saucers, a tour of his garden, his with woodpile., his sawmill, all equipped with ancient tools and machines using only the fuel and power of the human hand.

And his cabin.

One room.

With a trapdoor centrally opening to a container of space in the earth which he had carved out which served as his root cellar and his refrigerator.

And a two burner coal oil cook stove.

A leprechaun- like sleeping loft with a single agent mattress, woolen blankets and books lining the space, all ancient paperback cowboy novels, all which clearly had been read and reread many times over, on this Mountain, by the light of a coal tar lamp throughout through the whole of countless Berkshire nights. There was a tiny window from the vantage of his pillow which looked out into the forest and from which one could see the lights of Pittsfield twinkling in the distance.

Wow.

Bill Strong, even from this distant shore of life, our own days passing us like a tidal wave washing us like a tidal wave up to the far shore that you had reached when we knew you, the Taylor family still thanks you.

Thank you for sharing with us what is possible despite all of the gravitational pull of modernity against it, that life can be lived in utter simplicity if you have enough resolve, enough ingenuity, enough courage, enough strength.

Bill Strong died in Bed 1 of the Hillcrest Hospital Intensive Care Unit at the age of 78 after whispering to me his lips to my ear, "Thanks Dr., I think I have had enough." Despite the final stage nature of his congestive heart failure, he was able to manage a smile of peaceful acceptance as he with old left hand squeezed my young right hand as he took flight. My sense at the time was that his destination would look a lot like his Shangri-La on the hill, divine light and all.

A Final Examination

Mavis Hayes

Do not even know where to start.

Not that the recollection of our first encounter has faded a bit into memory over the 39 year interval since.

Our initial introduction took place on First Street. I am sitting at what we referred to as "Dr. Rubin's desk" which had been planted in the same position since 1949 and served as a Command Central for all operations -paperwork, phone calls, patient counseling all of which were profusely at hand. Most important lab results, x-ray reports, back to work forms, etc. could be found somewhere in the haystack shaped paperwork sculpture, mixed in with a few tuna sandwich
   wrappers and Kleenex wads that may have been used for anything from grieving to clearing tuberculous bronchial secretions. Thank God for the moderate invention of waste baskets and laptop computers.

There was a comfortable sitting chair placed at the left side of the spacious old mahogany launching pad desk, from which uncountable life stories had year after year spewn forth -what do they say? Sex, Lies, and Videotape.

Mavis's story was not among the more forgettable.

It was mid-afternoon on a busy Friday. The finish line of 5 o'clock (means 7 o'clock) was in siight but with a busy waiting room of chattering patients (the Pittsfield version of the Buena Vista Social Club) finishing time was still like a hazy mirage in the desert. It was in the fullness of this chaos that Mavis sort of arrived like the marquis actress erupting onto stage midway through Act I of a theatrical production, the action pausing for audience approval and recognition of true star power. A star does not meander onto a stage. A star springs onto the stage - determined, resolute, confident, unique, charismatic.

Mavis was pre-announced by a distraught nurse with something like "There's a lady out here who insists on seeing you." Though Mavis had also burst into the conference room choosing to announce herself before the nurse could finish her sentence. I mumbled something to myself like,"You've got to be shitting me." Her strong suit was clearly a flair for the dramatic mixed with a minor in hutzpah all delivered with a grand flail of upper extremity gesticulations. Her couple of sizes too large grand chapeau angled with Lauren Bacall in mind, her mohair dress coat with fashionably cut lapels, and her suave shiny high heals all striking a strong impression of high style which belied the fact that under her coat she was adorned in a hospital johnnie with its little blue florets and loosely tied rear flaps.

You expected her to say something perhaps like "Well, helllooo dahlink .... " I invited her to take a seat (she already had) and let me know what was happening, though her story had already commenced. Apparently she had been a patient recently on 2 Jones, our local psych unit, actually about an hour before, for a few day stay and had ceased to find the accommodations fully satisfactory and at midday had placed a call to a local taxi service and had taken her leave. She stated that she had heard about me from someone and thought that we ought to talk.

"Well, why were you in the hospital?" "No idea." Just some vague summary dismissal of some idiot in her family thinking absurdly that she was completely crazy or whatever. Minor point. "Well, what can I do for you?" "Well for one thing you could have them send the rest of my clothes to my house and for another you could give me something for my nerves and may be something to help me sleep." And thus we were off to the races.

For a while we met every couple of weeks. She never missed a scheduled visit. She never arrived late. She was never not elegantly appointed in all ways including a coterie of colorful headwear, jewelry, and generously applied makeup, and usually with a wide smile with a bit too much perfume and lipstick. She would always arrive with an installment size dose of her life's story; we would spend some time reviewing a few physical symptoms, tweak her medications a bit and schedule a return visit.

Salient features of this picture included the account of ongoing struggle with depression, the need to continuously ward off plotting some way to end it all, long sleepless nights, the fact that no one in her family (some Anglo-Irish mixture with a trace of blue blood and some significant standards as to education and deportment) would talk to her, and the fact that her daily medical regimen was quite routinely set into solution chemically with a quarter or so of gin and tonic or dry vermouth or ginger and whiskey, depending of course on the season.

In the summer she would take off for a month or so for the high season in "Bah Hahba" where she would be the houseguest of some more peripheral family members who apparently found her delightful company. She looked forward greatly to those sojourns and always returned tan and relaxed, smiling much more for a while. I tried not to check her liver functions immediately upon her return.

This went on for a number of years and eventually we had gotten to know each other extremely well. She collected old time sheet music which she would often share an interesting edition of with me. We were often able to telescope visits into reasonably ordered vignettes into which I would wedge one brick at a time in editorial style building a case against her chain smoking of cigarettes and the continuous attempt to solubilize her problems with alcohol.

It was the last Friday of the year in the office; when the office closed that day late in December, darkness already having fallen by 4:30, we would all go home to our families for a Christmas holiday. Mavis was scheduled to be the last patient. She was lonely, clearly closer to the edge than usual (she usually wavered in a no man's land between schizoid and borderline, eyes red, swollen, tearful. The last patient always realizes they can talk pretty well as long as they want to.

I knew this was going to take a while as she launched into a detailed reenactment of her very early childhood, painting an image of a well to do Victorian appointed homestead with overstuffed furniture, thick carpets and drapes, old fireplaces, unfortunately the warmth and comfort of which were belied by the rageful temperament of her viciously crazy alcoholic Irish mother. She proceeded slowly into and through this story, now at 60 but now back in the 3-year old little girl's body being tormented by her vindictive mother, the details of each snarl, each vulgar epithet unfolding in sequence rising into a crescendo and a shriek, "she ...." the words indecipherable on her lips.

"And she said what?" And she said, "She ppppushed me into the oven."

We both broke into tearful exhaustion and embraced as she wept for about 20 minutes, her head on my right shoulder.

We collected ourselves. Her makeup had been baptismally ensanguined. And I saw her face for the very first time, with wrinkles and the erosions of a lifetime of living with the fear of annihilation, asphyxiation, or death by strangulation. On her face there was a quieted expression of peaceful surrender which she was then able to maintain for an interval which ironically given the tortured in perpetuity nature of her personal war was not able to be rewarded with an era of peace of equal duration.

One year later she showed up with a spiculated irregular nodule -a crab- on chest X-ray and she was dead three months later. We were unfortunately never able to reach our own closure, reflect on her journey, or say goodbye given the man overboard nature of her final illness.

But the cancer did bring her to the absolute release that she had always sought in her own beautiful and unique way, both glamorous and not. It was as if she had finally done that which had come here to do.

Joseph Ancora

I just had a massage.

Emily and Mark and Cindy and I are reclused in the mountains of North Carolina. We are at an F. Scott Fitzgerald spa carved out of the side of a mountain with a ten mile view. It is constructed and appointed in the style of Frank Lloyd Wright with an interior appointed with a myriad of mission oak accoutrements. A million ancient stones have been constituted to form the exterior, fountains, caverns, tunnels, pools, all carved out of the side of a mountain but reconstituted here for the long run.

Cindy and I just had a "couple's massage," our first though over the years I have had some memorable massage experiences and seen many other similar awe-inspiring landscapes, and have developed a taste for various of life's luxury items. The taste appeal of caviar is not beyond my appreciation, I love sweetbreads sautéed in white wine, and the elegance of morning coffee (cinnamon Italian roast), evening Red Sox games, and long snuggling nights in our sleigh bed with Cindy all suit me fine.

I have one more chapter to compose for this memoir; I want to write about all of my children and how they fit into this dreamer's country doctor's journey, how that it has been all about and for what I see in them.

The only other remaining slice is to write down some very personal thoughts on my friend Joe Ancora, who sadly left before being able to enjoy these desserts of life which we reserve for the sunset. It is not an accident that I saved him for last. Thinking back on our times together is a bittersweet process. It has taken some time to be ready.

In the words of Bob Dylan, "He was a friend of mine."

Joe and I also had our first introduction on First St. We are both about twenty five years of age at the time and had an easy likeability with each other. He seemed to have already known me well for reasons which I can only attribute to the cosmic realm. I treated him for asthma. He wheezed like crazy at that time and often required steroid interventions. Albuterol had not yet been discovered. I spent some time explaining that his habitual use of cigarettes was greatly ill-advised given the severity of his asthmatic symptoms. This had a positive yield when not many years later he quit smoking for the long run.

After that my relationship with him was mostly as a satisfied customer. Joe played the piano. In fact in the Berkshires he was known by the moniker "Piano Joe" and anyone who was not familiar with his musical abilities had been living under a rock since Moses was a pup. Cindy and I always loved getting out for some fun, especially if it involved music, especially if it involved the piano, and especially if it involved Joe.

The story goes that his Mom noticed when he sat down at a piano at kindergarten age; he gave the appearance of having had lessons for a number of years. Not the case. It had to have been instilled from a previous incarnation. By eight years of age his parents had signed him up with Hammond Organ Company to sit on a stage in shopping malls across New England to hit the ivories for a fee. He was irresistible cute, ever so tiny, curly blonde locked, and could play like a banshee. By high school this evolved into being the frontispiece of a series of musical combos performing regionally to enthusiastic audiences. The music was selected on the basis of Joe's uncanny gift to duplicate almost any national performer - Elvis Presley, Willie Nelson, Ray Charles, Fats Domino, Neil Diamond, even Kermit the Frog. His Jerry Lee Lewis, especially Great Balls of Fire, was a showstopper guaranteed to bring down the house with the original Killer's version unadulterated. He could was the Great American Songbook incarnate, wrote extensive ballads and theme music of his own which he never seemed to play the same way twice. He claimed with all modesty to know about 5,000 songs pat, (I never requested a song which he did not know and claimed to not read a note of music or know one key signature from another.

Once I asked him what he thought of Gershwin's Rhapsody in Blue and he reported that he had never really listened to it but he returned the following Thursday afternoon, my afternoon off when we would often hang out and play with music, and proceeded to play all five movements of what many musicologists consider to be the greatest piece of American music flawlessly without a written note. Jazz, classical, hard rock, whatever, he owned it.

His prodigious musicality was sadly stolen from other parts of his brain usually given to standard academics. He was seriously dyslexic and found school a miserable experience from which he dropped out of in ninth grade. We would sit for long hours at our kitchen table and work on elementary math and English while the kids worked on their homework with the goal of gaining a GED but this never came to fruition.

So we knew him for some years as a jazz and pop impresario where he would sit behind a piano and play whatever people asked for plus a skein of his own unique interpretations that could take an audience from frenzy to trance.

The next interaction of a medical nature which I had with him came about ten years after our initial meeting. At that time our practice maintained a regular census quota on the local "McGhee Unit," our acute care substance abuse treatment facility.

On one Monday morning the head nurse handed me a chart with his name on it and told me, "He said you were his doctor." It was sort of like Thoreau being visited by Ralph Waldo Emerson and responding to the question "What are you doing in there?" with "What are you doing out there?" Actually he never before, during or after my own days of taking a drink and not taking a drink ever raised the issue of my own stuff.

Nevertheless it emerged that as a part of his professional career and playing environment he had been mired in since about the age of twelve, he had been consuming alcohol in massive dosage and never quit. Likewise the acceleration of his dosage had never waned until he had peaked out at about two quarts of Canadian Club with each evening's jam which the customer's loved, the proprietors loved, and Joe did not disdain himself.

We talked about the fact that this was probably going to kill him soon but that there was a viable alternative through the fellowship of a program called Alcoholics Anonymous. Joe never took another drink

He did work his way through some other stuff.

For about the next year he would run about ten or twenty miles a day. He did everything in a big way and had a lot of stuff to dump. He underwent extensive interpersonal counseling examining the complex nature of his life's saga to that point as to why he might have been at risk for alcoholism from the get-go.

He was soon back to performing again and played as well as ever. Occasionally drinking customers would offer him drinks and when he declined they would often push with "Oh, that's right. You can't drink." He would smile back with his wonderful, beautiful Joe smile, filled with wisdom and memory: "Oh, I can drink all right. But today I choose not to drink." And he never did.

Our personal relationship from that point also only deepened, I think largely on the anvil of the disease of alcoholism or perhaps more accurately the altar of recovery.

He had already become a fixture part of our family. Lacking family of his own, Cindy and I invited him to join us for our Thanksgivings back about when the Pilgrims were partying with the Indians. The post-turkey ritual of Joe playing and singing and our entire family including aunts, uncles, cousins, grandmas, grandpas singing our hearts out until about three in the morning had long become the fountainhead of Taylor family uniqueness - those times were so much fun, so heartfelt, so meaningful that the routine became ordinated as the touchstone for every major celebration, every major holiday, every graduation. Songs like Wind Beneath My wings, Over the Rainbow, Imagine, Great Balls of Fire, and too many to count became canonized as our family's anthems. When Joe played Leroy Brown, Grandma Long was expected to take center stage to boogie down, I mean down. Then of course there were the Taylor-Stalker Gospel Singers who I can vouch for saving many souls in need. Joe would play a special song for each of us. We marked Dad Long's passing with Willow Weep for Me which will always bring his memory to each of us, greatly thanks to Joe.

Some stomping was done. And a lot of laughing. And many hugs, and many tears.

We all loved Joe who would just play his heart out for all of us and had the minstrel's genius for extracting from each of us our best selves. Shy people would sing heart wrenching solos.

Awkward white folks would put on hats from remote third world countries and do amazing amalgamations of hula. cha cha, and Michael Jackson. All to standing room only applause.

Those were good times, maybe the best.

The closest I have seen in my own life to the full epitome of what family can be and mean.

Over the same years our medical relationship continued to deepen as Joe continued in his relentless process of adding fatal disease to his medical resume. As his twenty years of alcohol abuse became tempered by a profound and inspired recovery, he also developed Type I Diabetes Mellitus with nary missing a step. He applied himself to this and was able to control it effectively most of the time, learning to monitor his glucose levels closely and adjusting his insulin dosage. It was not long after that had been incorporated into his lifestyle when he developed myelofibrosis, usually a condition an individual can live with for a long time. Joe's case was viciously aggressive despite hematology/oncology support.

I saw him once a month for the twenty-five years of his sobriety. During those hours our relationship was purely doctor-patient. We took care of business. The nurses knew to book him for an hour interval. The largest portion of the time was used piecing together the shattered glass of his life gone by, his three marriages and his two daughters, his mother Rose who also became a fixture at family events, a 90 pound Nun of Intercession, don't ask. We discussed his living circumstances, family and work matters including working and living in the convent and caretaking the nuns which also gave him transportation. And his many years of travel, his transgressions, and his many victories. Happily for this quarter century he became a paragon in our local AA community. He knew and understood the steps and practiced them all religiously, sponsoring legions of "new alcoholics" of all ages. I repeat that for the many decade of our close friendship including about fifteen years when I might take a drink and fifteen years when I absolutely would not, he never even nudged at my opinion on alcohol vis a vis myself. Joe, wherever you are now, know that I greatly prefer the latter state, just as yourself, but I don't doubt that we both always knew that.

His latter years were also happily punctuated by the first long term successful romance of his life - Debra proved to be the true love of his life. Apparently she had fallen in love with him as a teenager "in the neighborhood" many years before but had never gotten up the nerve. They had some wonderful years together. She was an amazing advocate.

His health situation did not improve however.

Myelofibrosis, a disease that should not have killed him, din in fact, for lack of a bone marrow donor, at a youthful, playful, handsome charming young age of sixty, still able to play the piano as well as anyone I had ever seen.

When he passed I was visiting a daughter in California and not able to be present for his final days. I regret that though it was likely meant to be. Fate will have its way. The people who assumed that we were brothers were entirely correct.

I would like these recollections to be a eulogy of sorts for him.

Why do my feelings for Joe Ancora remain so deeply instilled?

My relationship with him as a patient was as protracted and technically complicated as anyone I ever cared for - fascinating, challenging, emotionally, physically, spiritually exhausting, but in the end the grand stuff doctoring is made of.

My relationship with him as a friend was equally profound. We both loved tunes with passion; we both loved the size, shape, contour of every set of 88 keys we ever saw or touched.

We both loved and were loved by every heart and soul in the Taylor family.

But in my heart of hearts I deep down believe that it was something entirely different.

From this very long view at which by the grace of God I have safely arrived it is my opinion that Joe Ancora from our first handshake knew me with a penetration of considerable aesthetic and spiritual awareness, knew me like the back of his own magical hand, and found me to be not wanting. A good and decent man who was able to love without question or qualification. And I know as well as I know anything that in the deepest humble recesses of my own soul that he always knew that I felt the same of him.

"Make sure you've got it all set to go,
before you come for my piano."

Jackson Browne

ROBERT M. TAYLOR MD

THE LAST GOODBYE

It was parsimoniously late on a Sunday afternoon,
the lateness of the day at one
with the lateness of the season,
the austerity of March resonating
with the cold stillness of the air,
winter still able to take a final bite,
like a steady old dog finishing its watch;
the solitude broken only by the rush of rising muddy waters,
flowing forcefully onward,
rising to fill the riverbed below,
below the little house at the foot of the hill,
the rush of water refusing to answer,
as only nature can refuse,
whether it was Winter or Spring,
or whether this was an end or a beginning,
but only that this family's world was pregnant with change,
and leaning toward labor.

Grandpa leaned against his well-worn broom,
the support much needed,
as his miniaturized frame which had served him loyally
across eight decades of walking to work
was now frail and bent
by the oxygen starvation mandated
by the stiffness and scarring of his lungs,
lips now painted with the darkness of venous blue.
His chore had been completed,
the wisp of snow across the few steps of sandstone sidewalk swept clean,
a task that seemed quaint but largely pointless,
to his grandson,
who now stood before his grandfather,

with his own agenda,
on his own schedule,
here for a weekend hug and goodby.

It would take until now,
it would take these four decades,
for him to know how much
his grandfather knew back then,
and why despite the infirmity and the dyspnea
the softness of a smile grimly traced its way
across the old man's countenance.
The tiny house
which had served as Scotland in America
for these flown by years,
which had yielded shelter, warmth, succor,
was soon to be departed from for the last time;
the ambulance would come
and these tired bones would be exited for their final care,
and for this, the passage should be made clear.

Yes there was wisdom in the elder's eyes
as he gazed upon his grandson,
and his young bride resplendently side by side;
wisdom, and some amusement, and much pride.
An unknown artist finishing a piece he had loved putting his hand to.
A poet finishing the last words of a verse and placing a period.
Amusement at the blue jeans and the work shirts
and the work boots and the wire-rimmed glasses
with which this fully American medical student and his glowing wife costumed
themselves,
the erst coal miner knowing much more of the history of work clothes
than these two who craved connection

with the decent humility of honest labor and laborers
and were willing to work themselves.
Pride at knowing that there was unashamed idealism in their demeanor
of which much good was certainly to come.
And both pride and amusement
at the ferocious passion with which these two
bound themselves to each other,
reminding him of his own young love,
in village Cowdenbeath in an earlier time now gone.
He knew the that this was a romance that would endure
the slings and arrows that were to come
and would climb the wall into a new century as a unity,
an indivisible force, a long enduring waltz.

All of this he knew as he stood now so long ago,
and held my young body firmly to his own,
aged heart and child's heart touching,
as he whispered into my right ear,
"Aye, Bobby, it's a comin' and a goin'."

I think of this now
because late Winter is coming again
and I am drawn to asking myself
as I am awash in the pool of singular kindnesses
which life has given me,
and weep with gratitude at the mystery and magic of it all,
the grandeur of the love between man and woman,
the fineness of astounding children,
the ecstasy of those children having lovers and children of their own,
the divine nature of this continuum,
the power and the might and the plan and the beauty
of this fast train coursing across old time.

I stand in awe of it all,
and say a humble prayer of thank you,

to those before me,
who made plain the way.

Aye, Grandpa, it's a comin' and a goin'.

11

MISCELLANEOUS

THE DEVIL IS in the details.

Pharyngitis.
Sinusitis.
Otitis media.
Otitis externa.
Conjunctivitis.
Laryngitis.
Bronchitis.
Tracheitis.
Pneumonitis.
Pancreatitis.
>Acute
>Chronic
>Chronic recurrent
>Acute recurring subchronic
>What ever
Hepatitis.
Descending cholangitis.
Diverticulitis.
Cholecystitis.

Spastic colitis.

Breast carcinoma.

Carcinoma of the prostate.

Carcinoma of the colon.

Bronchogenic carcinoma.

Merkel cell carcinoma.

Lymphoma.

Lymphosarcoma.

Myelofibrosis.

Fibromyalgia.

Osteoarthritis.

Rheumatoid arthritis.

Systemic lupus erythematosus.

Erythema multiforme.

Contact dermatitis.

Psoriasis.

Eczema.

Crotch rot.

Parkinsonism.

Amyotrophic lateral sclerosis.

Migraine.

Sleep disorder.

Sleep apnea.

Attention deficit disorder.

Somatization syndrome.

Menopause.

Perimenopause.

Erectile dysfunction.

Hypogonadism.

Pelvic inflammatory disease.

Sexually transmitted disease.

Gonorrhea.

Essential hypertension.

Renal failure.

Pyelonephritis.

Cystitis.

Nephrolithiasis.

Type 1 diabetes mellitus.

Type 2 diabetes mellitus.

Diabetic peripheral neuropathy.

Or as my associate Dr. Craig Kirby refers to what we do: Drips, moles and sore holes.

One fair question is whether or not a single physician can be competent in dealing with all of these issues.

And really, this is a partial list composed in two minutes off the cuff.

Well I never said that we did not always have a lot of help. And the feedback and recommendations of specialists and consultants also provides an ongoing continuing medical education process, which along with the Internet, a few journals, and the New York Times can keep a doctor pretty well up to date. That in addition to the fact that in this day and age there many conditions about which the fund of information is rapidly changing and massive and the currently afflicted person with these conditions should only be handled by a skilled specialist or often sub-specialist with the family doctor serving as backup to give support, and some interpreting, offer guidance.

But the converse is the typical hospital discharge plan whereupon a patient is discharged with a list of 7 diagnoses and 7 appointments with 7 different specialists to get to with 2 catheters, an indwelling IV, and a gastrostomy tube en tow. Isn't it easier to have them see their family doctor next Wednesday at 3 o'clock and have him sort out the necessities and priorities?

Generally this is a little more sane.

Anyway we do cover a lot of ground.

12

SPECIALISTS

By any other name

Specialists are doctors that develop an expertise in taking care of one particular part of the body or body system. Now basically all doctors are specialists, so we might just as well call specialists doctors as opposed to back in the day when doctors took care of everything.

A call I get commonly, once a week or so goes something like this. When other doctors call, the call is put through even if you are in a room with the patient. Though a specialist may call about anything-looking for information, comparing notes, being courteously informative, they often say something like, "Look, Mr. or Mrs. Jones really needs to do such and such (have a procedure, take a medicine, whatever) but he or she will not do it unless you talk to them. Which we promised to do.

There are two types of specialists who make these calls. Some understand that doctors in the process of dealing with all four arms and legs and such engender a special type of mutual trust with their patients and thinks this is a useful thing. Some, usually more cerebral, highly focused specialists with thicker glasses really see just the disease and do some type of sublimation process about it being attached to a person and do not really care why the patient will do whatever we tell them to do, they just want it to get done.

Both types serve wonderful purposes. The former type, I always thought might have made a good family doctor, the latter type not so much.

The entire mindset of being a Jack of all trades, Master of none has always been an inevitability for me, both my nemesis (asking the meaning of everything can be very time consuming and cumbersome) and my salvation. Pondering the interconnectedness of all things has led me to both my deepest awarenesses and by most severe exhaustions. Hopefully one or two good poems. And maybe a few healthier, happier patients.

13

MENTAL HEALTH ISSUES

Still Crazy After All These Years
PAUL SIMON

Crazy is as crazy does.
FORREST GUMP

Crazy As A Loon
JON PRINE

IF CLIMBING BEN Nevus is a good enough challenge for any serious hiker, then a general discussion of mental health issues as they play into the daily fray of the life of a family doctor constitutes Mt. Everest.

Grab your oxygen tank, invest in a really good tent, and fasten your seatbelt.

They say on Wall St. that if you want to churn a steady profit, invest in what you know.

Why don't we begin with depression.

As common as they day is long. All day, every day.

Capable of being fascinating.

The treatment especially with currently available modalities generally quite satisfying, though often only susceptible to stalemate.

Probably good to begin with the basic idea that depression has two faces, sort of like The Two Faces of Eve. There is endogenous depression (also known as chemical depression, or biological depression, or as bioaffective disease) the essence of which is that it essentially a neurochemical phenomenon which commonly occurs in our brains, especially common in those chromosomally programmed for a predisposition to the same. Then there is reactive depression (or situational, environmental, exogenous, etc.) essentially a not surprising psychological reaction to real life circumstances - illness, the loss of a job, a failed relationship, divorce, etc. Grief reactions are essentially a subset of this form which are hard to get through life without experiencing at one time or another.

Chemical Depressions are best treated with medication along with supportive counseling and adequate explanation and follow-up. Reactive depression can benefit from medication but more often the combination of counsel, support, and time will see the passing of the symptoms.

They both manifest with physical symptoms - weight loss or gain, sleep disorders, non-specific somatic symptoms, fatigue, weakness, anon - along with the conscious awareness of anger, loss, hopelessness, despair.

Simple, right?

Of course in the real world each depression is as unique as the given individual and usually some admixture of the two types which are best seen as occupying opposite ends of a broad spectrum maybe with a bell shape. I have many times made an initial mis-assessment as to type.

Here is a great simple handle once proffered to me by a psychiatry instructor, Dr. David Raskin, member in good standing of our local Mental Health Provider Hall of Fame if we had one, actually human being extraordinaire as I recall his life and work - a gifted healer.

Here's the pearl.

Depression equals loss.

Anxiety equals fear.

I cannot exaggerate the number of times those simple paradigms have helped me sniff out the salient underlying issues which the depression or anxiety in the mind of a patient was just trying to lead them to dealing with some feelings which they were unaware of or indifferent to.

I haven't even mentioned yet that depression and anxiety are first cousins and almost always occur in some interwoven pattern with each other and must often be treated in concert even though their treatment modalities can often interact or conflict.

To say that the pain of emotional strife dwarfs physical pain is a greatly under-valued truism which caring physicians should frequently remind themselves of if life doesn't do it for them.

Jessica Johnston recently turned fifty years of age. I have known her since when was thirteen. She comes from a severely dysfunctional family. Her mother though an intelligent and seemingly aware individual was basically exhausted in the process of single parenting her six children all of whom went a little off the radar. No one in charge noticed that this family in need of a scapegoat chose Jessica as a logical candidate and proceeded to victimize her through her childhood in every possible way, including her mother (also a patient) who in her own overwhelmed way seemed to need this dynamic. By the end of adolescence Jessica was often overtly suicidal and has remained so at least at intervals since. Over these four decades I have seen her approximately once a month in a role that combines some doctoring, some friending, some mothering, some fathering, some pharmacologizing, some comedying, At times the pleas of persuasion at warding off suicidal ideation have been like trying to play improvisational jazz with every word you know. Only a fortunate series of significant other relationships (usually not romantic, more likely a niece she is fond of, or a boyfriend's daughter, usually as I think of it a needy young female child). Surprise. I do not believe I have ever seen her not dressed in some form of Walt Disney paraphernalia of which she has amassed a rather extensive collection. Disneyworld for her is the counter-reality which has enabled her to live with and in this much more lacking daily reality. I believe she is happier now, and functioning more effectively, and with less of a threat of the suicide option than at any time in her life. I have come to know hew on a soul level and find myself deeply appreciative of her own basic goodness and willingness to do just about any kindness for others.

I have some personal experience with depression.

Somewhere around the midpoint of life after treading water for a number of years, mostly triggered some family of origin issues, after self-treating for many years with the challenges and rewards of husbanding and parenting, self-medicating with a whole lot of doctoring and a little Chardonnay, the bubble broke and I really couldn't pretend that things were okay any longer.

In my own case there is plenty of precedent in my likely DNA constellation judging from my first degree relative's tendencies though most of the turning of everything gray from the vivid black and white that I had always enjoyed was situational. At that time I ended up spending some quality time with three different psychotherapists.

Bob Sykes, PHD, marathon runner, beekeeper, alternative school progenitor met with me in a series of two hour sessions each of which felt like about five minutes. He drained my abscess.

After these few weeks, however, he pronounced me cured, which was much to my surprise. He was in a situation where he needed to get on to some more acute crisis. I will always be grateful for his help in learning that I could be helped as easily as I could help. People who know me would get that.

So I called up Mary Tierney who took on the mantle of Mother Number Two and walked me through my childhood one chapter at a time and then one issue at a time through my life's quandaries following which I felt a whole hell of a lot better. Thank you both from the bottom of my heart.

A few years later I think after slipping of the white wine banana peel I had a number of sessions with therapist Number Three, Verna, a pretty steady weekly date for a number of months, which were helpful and not uninteresting. She had this uncanny way when triggered by some wandering verbal didacticism or hypothetical intellectualized windy waft of verbal denial by interrupting me with her sardonic voice rising to a steep crescendo as in "Doctooooooooor!!!." This did more to free me from my previously perfected indifference to my skillfully plied bullshit about myself than anything I had otherwise encountered.

She sort of cured me, don't you think? Don't you think? Hey!

When I am attempting to encourage a patient much in need of therapy or some form of counseling services but showing fear or reluctance, sharing that without Bob or Mary or Verna I might be drooling or seizuring while talking to them can break down that barrier.

I guess if I were allowed to make one statement about depressive illness over my career it would be that the world of depression can be divided up into pre- and post-Prozac, and of course its progeny.

It is good for a clinician to always write a prescription after a thorough consideration of all alternatives but the vision of life without serotonin uptake inhibitors is a truly bitter pill.

Anxiety equals fear.

Which makes it so much easier to get to the bottom of phobias, self-treatment of every description, sleep issues, headaches of every description, irritable bowel symptoms, obsessions, compulsions, etc. With good targeting and probing questions in the context of good doctor-patient trust and a prescription or two a family doctor can help greatly with anxiety and often overt panic. Some individuals were born anxious and always will be but a great many others can grow beyond their anxieties or at least learn to manage them.

So it seems on balance that the whole of us spend most of our lives moments and hours in search of some sweet spot between too anxious and too laid back, just sort of mellow but awake, alert, sort of an emotional center cut. This of course in the ideal also has to be juxtaposed with a cross current of the depression spectrum, certainly not in the doldrums but careful, not too euphoric - this might disturb the neighbors - just sort of with the program but carefully avoiding anything overly enthusiastic or too exuberant, definitely if you around a lot of white protestants. The sweet spot. I think I actually found that spot once, as I recall maybe out on Chappaquiddick in midsummer with an all blue sky and a temperature stuck between 79 and 81 with the kids building a sand castle and Cindy and I just knocking through the Times crossword. Unfortunately I couldn't quite hold it.

Reminds me of an Archie comic cartoon I read once in sixth grade or so which gave me a big kick. Jughead was like drifting off in class and the math teacher alerted him from his slumbers by asking him if he was able to explain Einstein's theory of relativity. Jughead's response was absolutely he could but right at that moment he had forgotten it. The teacher's response, of course, was oh Jughead how unfortunate, especially since there are only seven mathematicians in the world who are actually considered to understand it.

So that's basically how one might look at how we deal with the great unwashed masses, i.e. most of us, the walking wounded,

There is also of course the rather infinitely broad spectrum of what we refer to as higher order mental illnesses referring to the DSM stratification of what constitutes saying goodbye to reality, waving back from a distance, and occasionally sending home a greeting card.

Most of the disorders involving potential for true psychosis are managed primarily through the psychiatric establishment, generally with good success and great expertise, especially if one factors in reasonable expectations and the finite nature of resources.

Most of these conditions are hard-wired - schizoaffective disease, bipolar disease with all of its ever-changing and complex stratification of subcategories, not to mention the more manageable OCD, ADD, ADHD, etc. Being primarily neurobiologically mediated, treatment is primarily psychopharmacological in the context of huge social support and care systems.

Family doctors tend to play a supportive role in this area, providing the best possible general medical care, and occasionally being able to offer some helpful observations or assistance on the basis of personal familiarity with a given individual or their family. And generally we are able to manage the milder cases of most of these especially once they are officially diagnosed and stabilized. Usually this is not overly difficult and is often just incidental.

There is no doubt that it will not be an extremely long time before we are able to do a lot more for these heartbreakingly suffering human beings, and then will look back at what we do now as even primitive. Thus is paved the path of medical progress.

In a couple of days I am going to read back through these last few chapters and I don't doubt that something will already have become quaintly out of date. If you can say one thing about the locomotive of medical care charging through time and the great plains of muchos disease it is that it is a ceaselessly fascinating ride but one on which you better take a firm grip and hang on for dear life.

The role played by all manner of mental health issues in creating daily challenge and mind-bending work for a practicing physician is not short of immense. An immense source of consternation and frequently a wellspring of professional satisfaction.

The War on Terror

It is August 22, 1968.

The highest sun of this particular summer day has long passed,
marched across, trampled by the relentlessly onward ticking of time.

One more inevitable revolution
of this ten billion times superannuated orb,
three hundred and sixty-five and one quarter spins per circumlocution,
to our knowledge without caring or ceasing.

An infinity of moments,
all much the same
as we slide in out of
the shiny Magritte night lit streets of this University town,
immersed in the slightly distant chatter and laughter of hanging out students.

Time may be the only unceasing dimension
but the memory of a given moment can be frozen forever.

We watch him on television,
protected by the signatured hotel podium,
exuding youthful vigor,
brilliantly articulating the dreams of our generation
which we had come to amass under the common umbrella
of End the War - Peace, Love, and Understanding.

Raising his right arm into the air
and flashing the Churchill V

which we had coopted as a sign of unity,
in the shared passion for smashing the weapons of war into plowshares.

"And now it is on to Chicago and let's win there."

Jesus, Billy Budd, John the Baptist, Joan of Arc,
the embodiment of the peace that was to come.

Moments later he was to lie in a pool of his own blood,
the unreplaceable cortex of his brain
punctured by a nidus of lead propelled from a hand held revolver
the bullet taken dead aim at the fineness of his mind,
his remarkable capacity for right thoughts,
the seat of his compassion,
the domicile of his intellect,
the heart of his enlightenment ripped away, shredded
by Sirhan Sirhan,
previously nameless,
twisted, alienated, lost in time and space Palestinian immigrant,
his own brain a scattered deranged vile carnage,
the prototype of what eventually we would come to know
as a suicide bomber.

The age or terror is given birth.

Hail Mary, Mother of God.
Blessed be the fruit of thy womb.
Blessed art thou amongst women.

What remains of that moment in me now
across a two generation span of moments,

toils, confusions, leavings, learnings,
four decades of celestial orbitings,
what remains is the horror,
the sudden descent from a pinnacle moment of rapture
into the vastness of the abyss,
paradise lost,
the before and after nucleus of my own so quickly passed journey.

We embraced, all of us,
the love of my life,
there as she was again and again yet to be,
there to catch my fall from the precipice,
and friends, indelibly imprinted friends;
the whole of a generation embraced in shared grief.

"Some men dream of things that never were and ask 'Why not?'"

It is December 6, 1980.
My steps across the parsonage lawn are no more or less hurried
than on any other go to work weekday,
stethoscope thrown over my shoulder,
hair longer than the no necktie collar,
bell bottomed, cowboy booted country doctor,
probably amusing to the ghost of the old Doctor Worthington
who had lived in this richly hearthed village house two centuries before.

The young doctor's accoutrements were residual evidenciaries
of the embattlements of bygone travels,
the length of the hair in particular an ongoing testimony
to four heroic musicians from motherland Liverpool

who had helped us all to survive,
who had delivered to us the strength to rediscover hope, healing, and joy
in the darkest of times.

Medical school had been traversed,
baptizing me into the robes of the shaman,
the marriage of our hearts had been codified,
I had become a father,
entrusted by God to share in the care of his angels,
Marie, the baby, born in the birthing bedroom above and behind my left shoulder
as I boarded our traveled Volkswagen van,
just going to work one more day,
rounds to be made, the aging and ill to be tended,
looking forward to the returning to this happy home
when darkness had returned at day's end,
the beckoning red and green of solstice rapidly approaching.

My life was not without its happinesses, its fulfillments, its meanings.

The dashboard radio announced:

"Last evening John Lennon, the former Beatle, was fatally shot
as he returned from a late night recording session to the Dakota,
his home in New York City.
He was transported by ambulance to Lenox Hill Hospital.
Emergency life-saving procedures were unsuccessfully attempted,
and he was pronounced dead."

I am paralyzed by the shock.
I stagger in disbelief back to our big blue shelter from the storm,
and embrace my family as the phone conflagration erupts,
the generation of love reaching out to inform itself,
trained for this,

strangely secure in each other,
secure in our beliefs.
We threw out a vast net of solidarity,
as John, now poet to the ages, would have wanted.
This pain was a process
in which we had been well-schooled.

Domini nobiscum veritas.
May the truth be with you
and may the truth set you free.

Secure in and untroubled by the knowledge
that the prophets of love,
the wagers of peace,
those who dream of revolutions of forgiveness,
those who are willing to Imagine,
must somehow be the first to go.

I return soberly to the VW van,
turn the key,
and go to work.

And one more generation passes,
seven thousand nine hundred and eleven more loyal turns of the globe.
The golden vivid morning sun of another September day slants
through the windows of my offices,
as I am engaged in the room to room chore of doctoring
as I have now known it to be for thirty years-
humoring, assessing, considering, persuading,
nurturing, supporting, crying for, crying with,
Scotch tape, Elmer's glue, an occasional Rubik's cube.

"Someone has flown a plane into the World Trade Center,
some nut I think," I am told as I enter the next room.

When I re-emerge a few moments later,
the last of the naiveté I am destined to know for this incarnation,
will have been dispelled.

I am told that the nut had some friends.

It is September 11, 2001,
and the world has changed.

We are at war,
again.

We, all of us, contact first our loved ones,
establish safety,
and then entrench,
dig into the electronic bunkers from which we do battle.

How can I help, who can I help.

This particular vision of hell is without precedent,
the magnitude of the devastation is grotesque,
an ocean of innocent souls set adrift
into a foul nebula of soot, a chemicalized incendiary.
The grand towers of civilization vaporized into particulate detritus,
countless human corpora devoured in the blast like insignificant debris.
A thunderous collision of opposite cultures,
a pot brought to boil across the eons of time,
fully armed B52's cast into a flight plan
from which they cannot be called back.

Alaahu Akbar.
Alaahu Akbar.
Alaahu Akbar.

The City,
the embodiment of the eventual hope of peace,
the Newer World that Bobby envisioned,
the loving world that John imagined,
these streets teeming with those
called forth from all the lands to be newly at home,
to struggle, to ascend, to labor, to want to be,
to compose, to create, to invent, to equilibrate,
the ultimate and true symbol of a just future is pierced,
my city,
impaled upon a sword of evil hatred,
to the devil's extreme delight.

Time takes no pause.
There is no hesitation.
The heroes rush into the fires, dive into the morass,
willing to offer up life for life,
unquestioningly,
the world amasses itself and moves on.

This will not stand.
The whole of civilization
consecrated by this abomination
re-dedicates itself without pause
that this will not be.

We reclaim the immediate,
and have continued to do so,

and still do now,
as I stand on this museum's roof deck,
and experience this art.
This work is the creation of Cai Guo-Qiang.
He was born in Quanzhou City, Fujian Province, China.
He was twenty-three years of age when John Lennon was murdered,
and his vision depicts the limitless potential of man's inhumanity to man,
the full spectrum and ramifications of which
his own culture has a far longer memory.
Clear Sky Black Cloud.

Tears appear across my eyes and my heartbeat quickens
as I incorporate this sculpted out reenactment
of the rape of my surrogate mother this city
to which I have in my time borne witness.

And yet I also feel a deep spring of peace in my heart
knowing that this theater is acted out on a stage
surrounded by the skylined skyscrapered greeneried pulsating mass
of this intact and ongoing city,
trudging onward with new ideas, new births, new words
and that within the walls of this same institution are contained
the many centuried testaments to the glories of mankind,
the ideas of the artists flowing freely and with great insight and beauty
when allowed to be at their most unencumbered best,
preserved and protected to feed future generations of dreamers.

Baruch Atta Adonai Eloheynu.
Melekh Ha-olam.
She-asa Nissim
La Avoteynu bayyim ha-hem.

We are still here.

We continue to crave for and eek out some unchanging morsels of truth.

My index finger is poised on this camera's eye, anxious to record.

My lips are moist with the desire to express, portray what I have learned.

My arms are open and ready to embrace in caring love.

Embrace the concept that there is glory and dignity in life in all of its forms,
from the awe provoking expanses of forests and oceans, deserts and stars,
to the complex vagaries and strivings of each individual human soul.

That though the differences between us
which when indulged can lead to fear and distrust,
violence and attack,
the similarities,
our need for respect,
our craving to be seen, acknowledged,
our passionate love for our own children
and their right to futures of their own
when unleashed
can lead to a brilliant symphony
of genius and diversity.
In a thousand languages, we all crave god.

Yes we are still here.
And we struggle along.

My own spins do gradually become more numbered
but as I gaze upon the vista of this city's heart
and reflect upon those now in the fray
I am content that the torch has been well-passed
and when I must take my rest
I feel that I will rest well,
knowing that in the longest run
our ugly capacity for hatred
will ultimately be made small by our love and kindness,
and that when asked by those I love
to give just one last kiss,
that it can always be found here,
amongst these hidden away pages.

I do not feel terror,
and I am not afraid.

What I want
is for each of us to love one another.

That will be enough
to one day take along.

Old men want to be rich,
and rich men want to be kings.
Any king that's satisfied,
never was that sort of thing.

Bruce Springsteen, Badlands

for my children,
December 2006

14

HOUSECALLS

DOCTORS DO NOT make house calls anymore.

That theme has rung through the hills since Dr. Rubin was in knickers.

What is true is that in most of our country's families, the infirm, and the elderly trying to make it at home despite medical challenges do have an incredible array of support services based on "visiting nurses "serving as lynchpin to enable that goal. The time, energy, and paperwork contributed by the family doctor, entirely unremunerated, is a necessary but invisible part of that patchwork.

But of course we do not make house calls anymore.

Though an hour spent two weeks ago with Dorothea Kennedy, my patient of 40 years is still fresh in my mind. Thea came to this country from Germany 70 years ago, auf Deutschland she would say. We just always got along. Anything I can say to her in my butchered Para-Deutsch which I can retrieve from two years of German in high school with Herr Finser has been enough to make her day. She gives extra points for effort and even the briefest reminder of conversational exchange in her homeland where most of her loved ones still abide as well as their children and grandchildren, Die Kinder. I always thought it was the homesickness that weighed on her along with her G. I. American husband's alcohol use, (? A good teacher) in addition to a couple of poorly selected genes of her own destined her toward the several decades of her own alcohol over-usage while raising quite successfully her American family including Gisela, nurse practitioner extraordinaire and Nick, chief radiologic technician at Berkshire Medical Center and the go to when a difficult procedure needs special skills. The drinking is long in the past. She is now 95 and just not able to mobilize to a doctor's office. Congestive heart failure is making its presence known which it so often does when more acute illnesses fail to answer the call preceding the sounds of the trumpets.

We basically needed to go over things with each other. I enjoyed our conversation greatly as she did point out the history of the various knick knacks appointing the massive trusty Germanic china hutch commanding her living room which was a microcosm of the old country, much as my own grandmother's living room was the briefest of trips to Edinburgh. I loved watching her recall the old days, brag about grandchildren, and laugh at my botched German responses as she reclined under a slightly oversized but very beautifully-rendered oil painting of a younger Thea Kennedy in full silk gown radiating youth even glamour, (? her wedding picture) the final breadth and scope of a lifetime well- lived in my view.

Then there was back at the other end my introduction to Ernest and Kathryn Roberts, after they called in response to a short Berkshire Eagle article reporting on my new partnership with Dr. Rubin. They had called requesting a house call. It was a new thought to me, not really seeing my skill set particularly useful in a non-clinical environment. The phone call included the address on **Mohegan Street. I** remember Ernie giving the instructions as if of course everyone knew it like the Boston Common, or Time Square., New York. Yep. 109. Okay.

I parked the car at the side of the bungalow on the gravel driveway, knocked, and was welcomed warmly at the door by Kathryn and Ernie and immediately thought on Dorothy entering Munchkinville. Neither of this leprechaun couple approached five feet in stature, even including their mutual unisex hairdos of thick bundles of snow white hair. It was clear at the outset that the visit ritual was to include sharing a cup of hot tea - the tea pot was already boiling. While the tea was prepared Ernie early gave me the cook's tour of this Roberts sanctum sanctorum all filled out in post and beam pine panels, all cut, trimmed, and set in place by Ernie's own hands somewhere back in the 1930s. I have not been on Mohegan Street lately but I suspect that the corner pieces of this domicile still stand square.

Brief physical examinations were conducted, "say ah ", etc., the blood pressure cuff serving like the portable communion cases the priests carry for such visits. We got on fine and they made me promise that I would bring pictures of my babies next time. Guys with long hair went way up in their opinion during my visit.

Upon departing the inevitable question of how much came up; Dr. Rubin had indicated to me that our house visit charge was $15. I blurted out - "Oh, 10 "which seemed reasonable to me. Ernest handed over a $10 bill which he went into the bedroom to retrieve from some cubby hole while Kathryn handed me a plastic baggy of homemade chocolate chip cookies. Neither knew that I would have gladly paid them 10 bucks for that visit. And how did she know that about twenty years later chocolate chip cookies would become my drug of choice?

This went on every couple of months for a few years until a point in time when the calls quit coming. Then about a year later I got a call from Ernest Junior, new to me, identifying himself as Ernie's son and relating to me that his folks were getting pretty confused and needed some kind of nursing home perhaps. I scheduled a family meeting to be held at the homestead and arrived to find the entire family surrounding the ancestral family table, below the ancient pine beams. Tea was poured but silence prevailed. The three sons, all Ernest knockoffs including thick shaggy heads of white hair. They were septuagenarians themselves and Mom and Dad had gotten into their mid-90's.

Ernest and Kathryn did not have to speak for the evident conclusion to be reached that the acuity of their orientation had dulled considerably. The harsh silence was finally broken after I had sat at the head of the table, encircled by this clan, mother and father and faithful boys and lifted both hands in question - "Well?" After a moment's pause, Ernest Sr. offered to speak first, in fact insisted. "I want to make one thing clear, (pause). I love this woman. (pointing to Kathryn) (pause). That is all I have to say."

Silence. We all talked and fairly easily put together a care plan which included services enough to provide safety and care for Ernest and Kathryn until they passed away in their own bed in the alcove bedroom, in the bed they had shared for 70 years, passing less than one year later.

I have often thought back to Ernest's position statement and the lack of response from his three loving sons and his college educated family doctor. I mean what else is there to say?

There have been many, many times through the years when those words have come to me in my own mind - moments of joy, moments of admiration, moments of pain and loss, moments of rapture through my own journey with Cindy - "I love that woman. That is all. "

On the subject of doctors making house calls one that always makes me chuckle was a visit on First Street to the second story of an old family boarding house where you can rent one room for a modest fee, probably a little less if you have your own hot plate. The metal frame bed, banged up dresser drawers and mildly mis-hung shaving mirror were included. This visit was at the invitation of the Pittsfield police in that someone needed to pronounce some guy by the name of Harry, no one seems to have known his last name. Apparently he had been a patient of Dr. Rubin's.

I recognized him despite his lateral pose of recumbency where he had been more than relaxed for at least a few days and indeed moribund. I also recognized him in that he had also been the ticket taker for many years at a local downtown theater, one of the many still open at that time, a couple of blocks from his abode. The other things I remember her from that visit, a new personal estimation of how many empty beer cans can be accumulated in a layered counter triangular position in one 12' x 18' space. The other finding was a stack of unopened mail on the tiny desk next to the bed, about a two foot stack, not ordered in any discernible fashion, approximately 90% of which appeared to be requests for payment from the offices of Drs. Rubin and Taylor. I still think about this stack of bills and the patient's attitude of indifference toward opening them especially when there might be a package store open within a block or two where resources could be put to better use. Whenever the subject of collections comes up at our office meetings I am generally in favor of moving ahead as quickly as possible to the next issue.

While on the macabre.

For most of my first decade in practice, Cindy and I lived at 13 Cliffwood St. which I am still in Lenox Village is referred to as the parsonage which it had been for about a century until during the Carter years' oil prices had climbed steeply contributing to maintenance costs of the old Village structure. We made the purchase of it and to the chagrin of a host of Village residents painted it a deep Colonial blue as opposed to the standard white with green shutters of the preceding seven or eight decades. We were confident that our modification was at least historically accurate. We called it Big Blue and proceeded to add to our family with Cindy giving birth to Marie in the middle bedroom on the second floor and rounding out our comple-ment by bringing home Emily from Ray Haling's birth center in Pittsfield to Big Blue in 1982. The house had originally been constructed in 1803 by a Dr. Robert Worthington according to his shingle which we found in the basement, and the horse-hair we found when we knocked out a wall in the rear in order to see the distance vista of Lenox mountain. And this was also confirmed by matching dates between the deed and the information at the Church on the Hill cemetery headstones located a few hundred yards away.

On Clifford Street which at that time had a fair number of toddlers scrambling around, a rite of passage for our own kids when they reached approximately kindergar-ten age was to walk up the block "to Minnie's " a spinster who lived three doors down with a past history largely confined to the realm of legend and rumor.

She did for many years in her old age command the neighborhood for long summer hours from an old crotchety wooden table chair which she would perch centrally in her front yard. She was something around 112 years of age. From some previous cerebro-vascular accident or some such her voice was a crackling incoherent snarl of blurred vagueness which only 2 or 3-year-olds could fully understand.

On one fall afternoon, a Thursday, my day off from the office, with rake in hand in casual clothes well-seasoned, I received a call from Dr. Robert Brown, Lenox chief medical officer, a pathologist, asking a favor. Apparently Minnie's presence had not been detected for a number of days and Bob wondered if I could make a house call. I agreed. Not that I was looking for work but I definitely had no excuse on the basis of location. I went down to Minnie's and with the assistance of the police broke into the front door's collection of locks and navigated the long narrow side hallway in search of herself. This route unfortunately was similar to the obstacle course they use in basic military training, using instead of land mines, mountains of empty cans of Jolly Green Giant creamed corn, the lattice work of cans being amalgamated together by reams of age old newsprint which I am certain on thorough perusal would yield a comprehensive history of American presidential politics since Franklin Delano Roosevelt. We did find Minnie and transferred her by ambulance to Hillcrest Hospital where she received several months of wound care before being placed in an extended care facility where she died a couple of years later.

Do doctors make house calls?

On that particular one my personal knowledge of rodentry I must say was greatly forwarded.

Finally one for the sports fans.

Similar to my visit to Harry's I was called in mid-evening by the Pittsfield Police in late spring time to pronounce as expired a lovely lately who had been a patient of mine for years, Margaret Harrison. The diagnostic part of the visit was far from difficult. What was difficult was that at that time one had to wait for the arrival of the funeral director before vacating the premises. This evening's visit unfortunately did coincide with tip off of a NBA playoff basketball game between the Boston Celtics and the Los Angeles Lakers, also known as Larry Bird versus Magic Johnson. Without actually verbalizing a single audible word, the police officer and I looked at each other questioningly, and flipped on the television while we waited for the arrival of said official, sharing the first half of the game with Margaret, until half-time when the undertaker just happened to make his appearance. The score was 44-44 at the half.

Doctors make housecalls.

15

THE DYSFUNCTIONAL FAMILY

THE SUBJECT OF the dysfunctional family has been written on profusely by far more trained and qualified dysfunctionologists (I have about sixty of their catchily named tomes on my own shelves and often direct a given patient to one or the other when screamingly appropriate), but what the heck, I'm out there dysfunctional enough to add own my own bit. Just a few thoughts.

Firstly, the obvious. It's a long stale jesting retort to the conversational use of the term "dysfunctional family" to respond with "Don't you just mean family?" Ha-ha. But like most overused truisms therein lies tons of truth which should be held on to firmly whether being a doctor/travel guide of a patient in an acute family crisis or even the long term type of quick sand or at home water- skiing through one's own family ebbs and flows. I'm going to keep reminding myself frequently and often, redundantly and repetitiously that yes, all families have dysfunctions - the idea makes it easier to maintain a cool facade while actually aghast, sort of like that bar they crush your crotch with when you get on a roller coaster. Seriously, families are collectives of individuals and until I finally like Mose wandering about in the desert for forty years come across a totally intact, fully enlightened and performing, well-adjusted and at all times appropriate co-citizen, I am going to keep my search for the perfect family on hold.

Having said that may I observe that helping families cope with their own unique vagaries is a central part of what a family doctor is called upon to do and actually often obliged to do even when not invited to the get-together.

In a direct way, the entity of family dysfunction stands front and center with immediate relevance in dealing with the more obviously appropriate diagnoses, the gamut of affective disorders perhaps most obviously, anxiety syndromes, every manner of depression etc. finding their roots in family dynamics the correction of which can aide dramatically in relieving the painful symptoms at hand. Then on the broadest level what malady, acute or chronic, is not experienced and strategized for recovery outside of the context of family realities. This can range from the overt like why is it that you are staying in a relationship where your partner gets drunk and belts you every Friday night just like your mother and her two sisters did (they might also be my patients) with your son skipping school and your daughter sexually active at fourteen to the more mundane like do you have someone to look after you at home after your discharge from the hospital, in reality an important question in this day and age of third party regulation, i.e. the meting out of home care by insurance companies and people get discharged from acute care with non-legible lists of 23 medications in that mixed language of Greek and Latin and tubes hanging out of two or three orifices.

I did promise at the beginning passionate digressions.

So family being the playing field on which our balls get kicked around in this soccer game of life, (careful), it is implicit that the practice of medicine should be a continuous vigilance as to the relevance and significance of the full panorama of the family experience, that is apropos everything.

Actually as I said the subject has been well discussed in many forms (isn't the same reality the basic building block of the world of literature?), so this is just in recognition of the importance of staying clued in to those always evolving dynamics. But I did have a couple of more specific thoughts.

The other day I found my mind wandering for some random reason to a particular image from early in my practice ("back on Fist St."), let's say a typical office visit with the Reilly family (alias). At that time they always traveled in a sort of pack, like out of Lady and the Tramp. Mary Margaret leading the troops, slightly haggard but not devoid of administrative competence or disciplinary rigor, reminiscent of General Patton. A moving target but receptive, enthusiastic, not without a willing humor, not without an obvious joy for and pride in the rest of the pack - four vagabond elementarians, traveling as one, except for the fact that Mark would be on the table, Michael would be under the table, Raymond would be on the shelf, and Dennis would be jugging 40 pound medical texts in the corner like a black jack dealer. Dad was some type of fictional character whose current location was less than specific but probably in proximity to some beer in a glass and definitely off the child rearing radar. His wife though was a tour de force and clearly signed on for the long haul, a force of nature fully committed to the raising of these four awesome Huckleberry Irish Finns or be fully committed in the process.

My admiration for this woman has never waned and I say this in that I saw her just two weeks ago and she is doing fine.

That's the point.

Move the clock forward thirty years and this woman looks exactly the same age, is ready with the same sardonic sense of humor, continues to provide wonderful care , now to needy aged in our community, and travels with friends frequently, often to the old sod. She never talks about it but I don't think she skips Mass often despite being pretty pissed at some of the church's failings.

The punch line is that Mark is a high level big pharma executive married to a brilliant and beautiful marathon running wife, Dennis has four kids as hyperactive and blond haired as he and his gang of four ever were and spends eons of time on the ball field of the season with his gang, Dennis is filling cavities and saving for his two kids ivy league educations, and Michael, well he still spends a lot of time under the table.

And more strangely yet Dad has been my patient for about ten years, has never had or appeared to want a drink over that time, seems to know the starting times at every golf course in Florida and is simply one hell of a nice guy totally likable and very proud indeed of his remarkable family. Like most of us, "Regrets, there've been a few" but also tons of happinesses.

A slightly long but hopefully accurate way of saying as the observation of an old doctor but maybe as a caution to a young doctor and as a gently reminder to us all, it ain't over til it's over.

Never presume that the most confusing, frustrating, exhausting, heart rendering circumstances that any of us may look into the jowls of today constitute a permanent state of affairs. As one rocker said, the road is long, with many a winding turn.

Family dysfunction might often look like a hopelessly tangled knot but in fact the family is relentlessly fluid and resilient.

Which brings me to my final observation.

The story just told magnified by some large if indefinite coefficient would constitute the story of my life and career as a doctor.

How can I not wonder at the strength and nature of the fibers that hold families together - a force of nature with infinite theme and rhapsodies. Think the whole of Beethoven's Symphonies. Though my experience enables me to be a validator of the power of this force, I would be at a loss to speculate on the intricacies of the counter-currents that explain the same scientifically.

I have this thought when I gaze on the new World Trade Center and wonder how it is that our best architects, engineers, constructioners can create this tower reaching into the sky like a prayer to God, designed for perpetuity and with enough space, passages, and resources for people like all of us to within this prayer act out our own roles in the international dialog of the sharing of this planet.

All I am saying is to never underestimate the capacity of any family to find resolution, resurrection, redemption, just as any of us as individuals carry within us the same hopes and promises.

And definitely never underestimate the Reilly's.

16

ON DEATH AND DYING

" THE DIAGNOSIS OF an incurable or fatal illness is not the time to let down on the patient's behalf; fatal illness is a challenge for thoughtful, inventive, aggressive attempts to better the patient's state to any degree possible. The physical effects of the illness must be modified and kept under control as effectively as possible and the patient's attitude must be sustained as effectively as possible throughout the illness through the instillation of hope, hope that is tempered by honesty.

Exercise clinical judgement - spend time with the patient; the amount of time spent with the patient should be proportionate not to how interesting the patient may be at a given point in time but rather to how much the patient needs you. Use sedative medication when sedative medication is needed and pain medication when pain is the problem, distinguishing between the two and using adequate dosage. Make changes in the treatment program along the way even if only minor in nature so as to demonstrate to the patient continuing interest and concern.

Follow up new complaints and do not slight on physical examination - this can be of therapeutic value in and of itself. Select the treatment which will allow the patient to live the most comfortably even if not necessarily for the longest time, and avoid heroic forms of treatment. The continuance of life is not nearly so important as the conclusion of life as free as possible from physical and emotional pain.

At a very practical level it can be of immense value to consciously arrive at a judgement of when death is at hand. This judgement obviously can not be a casual estimate and ideally should be made in consultation, but once it is arrived at, the patient should simply be allowed to die.

In the final analysis we must inevitable ask ourselves, "To what extent are we becoming more or less human?" As physicians we may never be returned to the role of omnipotent intermediary to the next world - that would not be allowed by our own sophistication or that of our patients.

Nevertheless we must reassert ourselves in making the distinction between what we are doing for our patients and what we are doing to them. To the extent which we expend ourselves as extensions of the medical machine, at the expense of supporting our patient, providing counsel and consolation, we will be less as physicians and less as human beings."

With a highly echogenic sense of surrealism, I quote myself from a presentation on this subject I made at our Medical Grand Rounds as an medical resident in 1973.

I do sort of wonder what was the distinction I was making between incurable and fatal but other than that I still agree largely with this ethos.

I also hope that to the best of my human capabilities I have put forth the effort needed to live out these beliefs. My memory is certainly overflowing with recollections of sitting with patients hand in hand so many times, revealing a dreaded diagnosis, explaining the lack of reversibility of a condition, helping a patient I have known and loved for often many years across the final threshold. Oh yes, I have seen the eyes of death manyfold.

My primary reflection on all of those experiences at this stage is a sense of gratitude for having been allowed to - allowed to share in those pinnacle moments of ultimate reality, painful but revealing, and definitely more of a gift from my patients to me than vice versa.

At such bedsides I have learned the most of what I think I know or at least believe about life's meanings, significances, perhaps even where we came from, where we go to, and why we were here.

I do not regret the process.

On the other hand there is good news here.

The above of course was written long before our current era - that is the era of hospice - hospice thinking, hospice services, hospice philosophy. Much of what I was trying to make a case for back in my incipient days has rather wonderfully come to pass.

Among the things which we are good at in our own day (as opposed to the prior approval system) is in fact identifying approaching end of life, not just malignant disease but chronic degenerative disease in all of its forms or sometimes just the inevitabilities of age itself. We have across our land an army of insightful, dedicated, and skilled medical professionals who do this work with great compassion and fulfilling results. It is a pleasure to be a part of the team with this people, including identifying and implementing services, supporting the patient throughout the journey, and offering whatever can be offered at the end. Death has in fact quite generally become a more friendly outcome in our time.

I dearly wish that was all there was to say.

While quoting something I wrote in my cowboy days sums up much of what I still feel about the subject, perhaps more importantly this chapter has come to need a Part Two.

Thus

On death and dying: part two.

Living Too Long.

Just as in our time we have participated in and borne witness to a major renaissance in end of life care and this has indeed been cross cultural work of the medical, the clerical, the philosophical, the patient, the progress of science has simultaneously created another monster, the size and shape of which chills me with fears for the future.

It has become harder to die. Not because of the lack of skilled professionals at hand to help us with the process when the time comes but because in this era of megaton antibiotics, heart rate and blood pressure lowering beta blockers, perhaps most dramatically of all cholesterol lowering statins in combination with more pervasive access to better nutrition, more exercise, better mental health services, better quality medical care, a situation has evolved where it can be hard to go on and grow old and even harder to get on with it and die.

Good or bad??

Both I am sure but also expensive, chaotic for social and cultural moray and tradition, challenging to rituals and institutions; as we live older and older we have no choice but to also re-negotiate our beliefs, values, and customs around the general sense of how long is a good long life and at what point is the effort of staying in the game of questionable value. We really have cured a dangerous number of diseases.

Either Marc Anthony or Brutus said "Death being a necessary end, will come when it will come," - look it up - but the quote makes me wonder if either or both of them were on Medicare, took Lipitor everyday, worked out at Nautilus, had a yearly physical and if they did would they still be eating fruit and drinking one glass of white wine a day in the Forum yet today.

So more seriously.

This is my thought and really the purpose of this chapter.

Sort of ironic that I am writing this chapter as sort of an after thought, having considered this all a done deal ready to stick in some drawer, but then deciding I had forgotten something.

It surprised me when this omission occurred while spending so much time everyday day forever speculating with my patients as I size them up, patch them up, glue them together - about what the heck does it all mean and how much time do we have to figure it out and pack a bag?

At any rate I would be of the opinion from this vantage after watching my whiskers traverse the full spectrum of a lifetime that the single most important, challenging, significant problem which besets our kind as we enter a future of unknown things yet to be dreamed of is coming to grips with the idea of the end of life being okay, that the cessation of cardiac and respiratory function maybe needs to become an entity of timed volition and acceptance, a transition over which we as individuals and families take part in the orchestration and nature of with peace, joy, and willful openness to whatever might follow, the fulfillment of the mysteries.

We need to cease looking at death as an enemy folks.

In my experience it has much more often been a friend.

Sort of like turning our swords into ploughshars and making peace with our enemies and insisting on leaving in a way that shows true gratitude for the wondrous miracle of the soil and the sun, the stars and the skies, the lovers and the loved ones that sustained our time here.

The fact that those words seem so very all right with me probably means I better finish this chapter at this point while it sounds like I'm resolved on the matter and let the campfire burn down.

THE CLOCK

Le Dorsay

Clock Gargantuan.

Is it you,

whispering,

is it you,

surreptitiously miming your secret knowings,

you

with your daunting appendages,

able to be seen beating along from afar

such that the bored one waiting,

his own extremities crossed and folded on granite bench,

his own crumpled Times cast aside,

can rest,

matching heartbeat for heartbeat,

and watch your own beautiful arms sweep ahead.

A FINAL EXAMINATION

Clock gargantuan,

holding court over these hallowed halls,

echoing the distant squeaks and chokings of trains long off into the night,

now presiding over the sculpted homages and prayerful canvases,

left to honor your relentless steps from then until now.

Clock gargantuan,

marking out time,

ever the more greedy,

in the accelerating pace of your theft,

ever grander,

in the finality of the dominion of your judgments,

and the depth of your wisdoms,

regale,

in the declaration of the vastness of your realm,

pedestaled above the frenzied throngs of our current already late steppings,

above us all to be wondered about, pondered,

just as one day each of us,

yes every one,

from some much lighter ethereal perch,

will sit and watch this blue and green orb awash in its misty haze,

turn and turn,

performing again the circular ballet,

which we have always called,

today.

17

FOUR DAUGHTERS

NO JOKE.

Yes, I have four daughters.

I don't intend to have a tombstone but you could put on it, "He had four daughters."

That fact alone has made my life worthwhile.

I see them as the ultimate gift of love from Cindy, also the gift of both of us to the world.

They say Ireland's gift to the world is its people.

Our gift to the world is our daughters.

The four happiest days in my life were

October 16, 1971 when Cindy gave birth to Amy Caroline.

January 22, 1974 when Cindy gave birth to Elizabeth Pearl.

March 5, 1978 when Cindy gave birth to Marie Susan.

September 23, 1982 when Cindy gave birth to Emily Catherine.

My Grandmother Bradley was a Caroline and Catherine.

My Mother and Grandpa Long's sister were Marie.

Cindy's Grandmother was Pearl.

Grandma Kate, my father's mother was Katherine.

We always wanted to have a Lilly. Probably it's a little late.

We started out wanting a raft of kids.

This particular raft proved awesome.

They are all beautiful.

Their smiles could light up a hemisphere.

Their love and loyalty for each other is a miracle of feminism and makes me thankful for people like Betty Friedan and Gloria Steinem and for the effect they had on people like Cynthia Taylor.

They are all deeply intelligent with thoughtful, inquisitive minds.

I have learned to be cautious in debate with any of them, especially on articles of fact.

They approach the world with profound respect for the differences and vicissitudes of their fellow men and women; they attempt to make change by being the change, and setting an example of their own behaviors. Thank you Barak for verbalizing what they have always been.

They look at life as to be experienced, investigated, explored, not to be feared, abstained from, or saved for later.

Amy has a voice that can melt honey. The depth of her intelligence seems limitless. She is a wise soul.

Liz has a heart the size of Wyoming and uses it. She finds the downtrodden before they need to find her. Her kindness is pure gold.

Marie has the most natural intuitiveness about people I have ever witnessed. Her artistic sensibilities, first evident on the floor at age two are amazing. She still owes me an apple.

Emily, who says she is the favorite, is a powerful force for change. She has made it her mission in life to spread the word through research, education, and political action the sacredness of the art of breastfeeding. Isn't that where it all begins?

They have all married husbands, Nick, Jeffrey, Andrew, and Mark whom I adore and am proud to have as part of my life. All four remain happily married, a parent's dream.

And Grandchildren.

Cullen Alexander, Antonia Rose, Addison Michael, Greer Frances, James Nicholas George, and our baby Rose Cynthia Marie. So far. I could write a book about any of these fourteen awesome kids.

Why do I end with this?

Because I am a family practitioner.

I was born to be.

I know that soon it will have run its course.

And know that these children have been God's gift to me for trying my best.

HANDEL ME WITH CARE

It is May 14, 1723;
the curtain rises at the King's Theatre in Haymarrket,
upon London;
the sopranos Francesca Cuzzoni and Marghuerita Durastanti,
supported in harmony by the castrati Senesino and Gaetano Behrenstadl
sound forth the rapturous premier of Flavio,
mythical King of Lombardy.
In the first row orchestra anxiously seated
is George Frederic Handel, aged 38,
now settled for awhile
on the banks of the Thames
alter childhood gestation f. Germany
and a number of prolific years composing in Italy.
It is a grand moment,
the earth trembles throughout and the struts of history writhe and quake.
Less ceremoniously it is only a matter of days hence
that another musician,
Johannes Sebastian Bach,
journeys from Vienna to Leipzig,
with his entourage of wife and thirteen children
where he will ultimately pass without subsequent relocation
some 17 years later,
after suffering a cerebral hemorrhage.
It was several months after his arrival in Leipzig
that he carved out
the
lime
to preside over the first public performance
of The Passion According to Saint John.
Flavio rightfully was unintimidated.
Simultaneously in the New World

patriotic Massachusetts colonists were being

whipped into a fervor by one Crispus Attucks,

a runaway slave and rebel leader;

all unfortunately were

subsequently slaughtered

in what came to be known as the n Massacre

by British troops,

perhaps Handelian cousins,

the absence of which from their homeland of course

made Flavia's assignation of Lotario to the rule of England

an even more unopposed task.

Nevertheless the nefarious Lombardy/Boston axis of

conquering and revolt

was thereby established.

Meanwhile in Philadelphia

a 17 year old Benjamin Franklin is said

to have accepted his first position in the printing industry,

a career choice of some portentous moment

to which even Handel must agree;

in 1775 after co-authoring the Declaration of Independence

Ben is to have said,

"either we shall all hang together

or assuredly we shall all hang separately.·

Guido, Emilia, Teodorata, Ugone, Lotalio and Vitige,

as well as many unnamed patrons in the audience,

could hardly but concur.

It is not without similar consequence to the Fate of Man

that one must note the somewhat parenthetical fact

that it was in 1723

that Adam Smith

the first great classical economist,

i.e. the father of modem economics,

was given birth to in Fife,

located snugly between

the Firth of Forth,

and the Firth of Tay,
no relation of course to the poet.

Concomitantly on the peninsula ultimately to become San Francisco,
the lands were ruled by
the Costanoan Indians
unhampered by the burden of encroaching European thought or insight,
were busy pursuing
in unimpeded fashion
their tribals customs and rituals.
It is only out of respect for temporal urgencies
that we leap now
to the year 1967,
a mere span of 244 years,
little of great epoch having transpired,
in the interim.
President Lyndon Baines Johnson
has just appointed Thurgood Marshall to the Supreme Court;
he is to be the first black Justice on that august body,
the same Mr. Marshall who in 1954
had written the opinion referred to as Brown vs. the Board of Education,
which resulted in the desegregation
of public schools.
And in 1967 the American civil rights leader.
Doctor Martin Luther King,
was to have declared
that transfer of wealth from rich to poor
was a natural requirement for "true social justice."

The following year he was assassinated.

Israel meanwhile was taking control
of the entire city of Jerusalem,

outing the last of the Jordanians from power.

The Beatles were busily imagining themselves on a boat on a river and conceiving of an existence in perpetuity in fields of strawberries.

In San Francisco tribal cultures once again reigned as the children of America in beads and feathers declared the Summer of Love.

And the Doors of course declared in song with cryptic eloquence that people are strange,
when you're a stranger,
a subject which King Flavio of course wrote the book on,
which brings me finally to my point.

Yes.

It was in fact in the year 1967
at the annual Handel Festival in Gottingen
that King Flavio,
my hero,
my alter ego,
he of the phosphorescent chartreuse
and pink high heels,
not one to labor endlessly in obscurity
without the benefit of an audience
once again rears his beautiful countenance
for his first performance in 244 years.

A simple fact not lost on me,
a fact which stirs my soul.

What of all these words
scratched out across these weathered pages,
scratched out by this poet hidden in my heart
this poet recently published for the first time.

Bury them!!

Very well, bury them!!
In drawers.

In scrapbooks.

In the attic, the cellar, bury them!

For eventually if truth be in these words
like a Phoenix from the ashes
in some future country,
in some future incarnation,
Flavio and I shall rise once again.

As Handel knew well,
it ain't over until the fat lady sings.

EPILOG

WELL THAT IS about enough.

If I needed to have my say, that is definitely enough.

And at this point I am pretty okay with it, thank you.

I posed the question at the outset here as to whether or not with the transformation of the relationship between doctor and patient from the lifetime of such relationships which I have known to let us say something different- less personal, less intimate, more mechanical, more technology mediated- were we losing something of value?

I clearly feel that it is so. I feel that I and my colleagues over a long venerably traditioned span have done some great doctoring; enough so to create some nostalgia for what once was.

I realize now that the few ounces of motivation that it took to collect these thoughts in this form came largely from the need to have a vehicle with which to mourn its passing.

I have also lived long enough to know that it is only natural for the future to depart from and evolve out of the past, that we come here for a brief continuum of time and then to pass a torch.

Cindy and I had the opportunity to attend on a Sunday afternoon recently at the Cathedral of St. John the Divine a rare public presentation of awards to a cadre of the world's leading peacemakers, the Dalai Llama being the featured officiant. During the open question and answer period a Columbia University PhD public health school Dean posed the question: "As we enter a modern age of rapidly expanding population numerical demographics in the context of a superimposable technologically dictated restraint and geopolitical and natural resource confluences, what can we expect to happen in terms of cause and effect on resource distribution demarcations and counterinflusions?"

Professors love to ask him questions like that.

The Dalai Llama turned his eyes into his vast soul in a deep moment of meditation reaching for his answer as not a pin dropped in the great Cathedral.

He then lifted his continence with his usual blissful smile and answered: "Well you should ask someone young that question. I am old and soon it will be Bye-Bye!" offering a gentle wave with the kindness and innocence of a toddler and the wisdom of a God.

Shakespeare did say "Brevity is the soul of wit."

I am well aware that the future has never tended to look a lot like the past.

And I am okay with that.

But I do invite the caregivers of the future to take a page or two from the past. I am reminded of a comment made by Jeanne-Claude quoting her husband Christo, both the creative geniuses of the Gates in Central Park, speaking at a consortium at the Metropolitan Museum shortly before the unfurling of that masterpiece. She was reflecting on their arrival in New York City from Italy many decades before, Cristo had taken her for the ferry ride across New York Harbor which Cindy and I have also embraced in rapture so many precious times. Christo said to Jeanne-Claude: "Do you like it? I give it to you. It is yours. " And that is that.

And as Calvin,

My alter ego, my role model,

said on his last go around,

"The days move slowly,

but the years just fly."

THE MIST

subtitle: a windy waffle

"Where do you go when you get to the end of your dream?"
Dan Fogelberg

What manner of journey this,
this exit, this departure,
this final unplugging
from the seemingly known vantages and dimensions
which have long prevailed with an apparent certainty
the final (or not) parting from every other mortal known,
cared for, cared about by, cried about by, cried over;

what manner of journey this,
unknown with bitter equality
to the myriads gone past
that threshold beyond physicality,
beyond that last feeble throb of myocardium,
that last synapse ignited,
thinking given disposition, movement suspended, energies set neutral;
unknown to the bygone king,
unknown to the duplicitous papal conniver,
unknown to his pure cousin at labor, loyal believer,
unknown to the thief, the surgeon, the babe,
the soldier fallen in battle, the swerving teen on the county highway,
the poet, the barker, the monk, the meek, the slave;

all left with the same goods, the same burdens, the same summons,
all equally and weightlessly alone,
yet on the wings of a single theory
of their own conceiving.

This is mine.

It is the earliest breath of awakening morning,
or if you prefer the last breath of a long ticking night,
a long night of wondering,
or worry or rapture or peace,
inevitably at end,
or more precisely
that miraculous open field of time between the two,
that golden wind caressed expanse of time
leading to the above,
liberated into timelessness.

And there is the mist,
infinite in its cool velvety softness,
soothing this newly birthed spirit,
as it glides onward, outward, into the beyond,
blurring but enhancing with a divine enlightenment
the final viewing of that very perfect scape
a last farewell to the magnificence of the earth.

The Hebrides, the rising sun, the continents,
the haze of the outer atmosphere,
do a gradual fade into past.

And there is sound,
the peaceful drone of tranquility,
a choir of mantras, melodies of the angels

singing happily for this going,
melodies known only to the undeparted
as perfect silence.

My own theory.
An arguable proposal, at best.

But what has come to interest me
as the days from my arrival upon this ultimate voyage shorten,
achieve imminence,
is the deepening knowledge
of the awesome flow of the river
that has carried me to this awaiting door.

The full splendor of all that has been seen and felt;
amazing, amazing, amazing my pitiable plea;
I must declare that I recognize, accept, embrace
the infinitude of this transpired life;
that I humbly beseech forgiveness for holding back,
for falling short, for a myriad of wrongs.
That I arrive here and then depart
with a heart richly laden with love given,
love received, love flowing in richness across these times.

Odysseus knew
that there is a difference between
a journey with an unrevealed destination,
that is,
not knowing where you are going,
or why,
and embarking on a journey
without knowing
where you have been,
what you are taking along,
what has been left behind.

I know.

That when I am gone,
though winds will continue to sweep loose snows
majestically off of the Eiger's pinnacle,
the towering peaks of the giant Sequoias
will continue to bloom upward to heaven,
the snow leopard will still wander Himalayan wilds
foraging for food, shelter -
life will continue in all of its ways.

But I also know
that in the hearts of those I have loved
an occasional thought will be of me,
and in that way, I will remain.
There will be an occasional smile,
an occasional story (exaggerated),
a random remembering sigh or tear,
perhaps something will be given,
a right cause struggled for.

And I know.

That when I have loved you,
and been loved by you,
this was real,
inviolate, beyond understanding,
but real and now ready
to be transported into what lies beyond,
and all that I came for,
and all that in the end,
I care to take,
is the rightness of that love.

Acknowlegements

I WOULD FIRST like to thank now passed Evelyn Hart for my portrait which she insisted upon creating from a photo after taking up drawing and discovering her talent and passion while grieving the loss of her dear husband Winston, whom she had previously described falling in love with sixty years before on the slopes of Bousquet when they only had a tow rope. She was a wonderful woman.

With all due sincerity, I would be remiss to not make note of the profound sense of gratitude which I carry close to my heart for the panoramic legion of patients over these many years who have entrusted me with their care and opened to me an engrossing window into the human soul. I especially thank those individuals mentioned in these pages, specifically, indirectly, or in composite and hope that this extended sharing may do others some positive service.

I would also like to express my infinite respect for the cadres of medical professionals whose work I have been so fortunate to bare witness to, especially the heroic legions of nursing professionals whose own work and wisdom the doctor is often credited with, and who likely know when we fail or succeed more accurately than we can judge ourselves.

Special appreciation to Family Practice Associates office managers Judy King and Patricia Masoero whose work and imagination helped create our entity and manager/ nurse/leader/and conscience Cynthia Iwanowicz R.N.who will hopefully one day grasp the vast scope of her personal contributions to our community.

And hopefully evident in the preceding pages a lifetime of gratitude to Cindy and our daughters for the wealth of patient tolerance of the intrusions into our home and personal lives which enabled me to pursue my passion.

And to Amy Caroline, Elizabeth Pearl, and Marie Susan for editing my life, and Emily Catherine for so diligently editing my book.

Made in the USA
Middletown, DE
08 April 2016